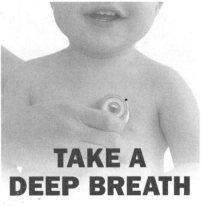

TAKE A
DEEP BREATH

Clear the Air for
the Health of Your Child

TAKE A
DEEP BREATH

Clear the Air for
the Health of Your Child

Nina Shapiro, MD

Director, Pediatric Ear, Nose, and Throat
Mattel Children's Hospital UCLA

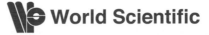

World Scientific

NEW JERSEY · LONDON · SINGAPORE · BEIJING · SHANGHAI · HONG KONG · TAIPEI · CHENNAI

Published by

World Scientific Publishing Co. Pte. Ltd.

5 Toh Tuck Link, Singapore 596224

USA office: 27 Warren Street, Suite 401-402, Hackensack, NJ 07601

UK office: 57 Shelton Street, Covent Garden, London WC2H 9HE

British Library Cataloguing-in-Publication Data
A catalogue record for this book is available from the British Library.

Cover photo courtesy of Getty images.
Author photo on the back cover courtesy of Reed Hutchinson.
Section two photo (p. 65) courtesy of Clare Bloomfield.
Section three photo (p. 137) courtesy of Photostock.

TAKE A DEEP BREATH
Clear the Air for the Health of Your Child

ISBN-13 978-981-4354-97-4 (pbk)
ISBN-10 981-4354-97-X (pbk)

Typeset by Stallion Press
Email: enquiries@stallionpress.com

Printed in the United States of America.

and more importantly, what not to worry about. *Take a Deep Breath* will undoubtedly set your mind at ease and help everyone breathe a little easier."

— Scott W. Cohen, MD, Pediatrician and Author of 'Eat, Sleep, Poop:
A Common Sense, Guide to Your Baby's First Year' and
co-founder of Beverly Hills Pediatrics

"*Take A Deep Breath* will keep parents from hyperventilating! It is the perfect hand-book of breathing written by an impeccable surgeon who is, first and foremost, a mom. If this book were required for every new parent, it would save pediatricians a lot of time and parents a lot of heartache."

— Cara Natterson, MD, Pediatrician and Author of 'Worry Proof:
A Pediatrician (and Mom) Explains Which Foods, Medicines, and
Chemicals to Avoid to Have Safe and Healthy Children'.

To my patients and their families,
of whose lives I am privileged
to be a part.

And to my family,
my breath of fresh air.

CONTENTS

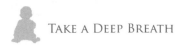

ACKNOWLEDGMENTS

There are so many people to whom I am grateful in making this book happen. First and foremost, I am grateful to my patients and their families. Many of them I meet only once or twice, for an office visit or hospital consultation. Others become part of our medical 'family', whether it's by virtue of treating their brothers or sisters, or by virtue of their needing our care for a lifelong chronic illness. In any scenario, parents trust me with their babies, which is the most monumental gift one can give. While medicine and surgery are hard work, it's harder to be a patient than it is to be a doctor.

I could not begin to care for these children without an amazing group of doctors and nurses with whom I am fortunate to work at UCLA. While I wish I could personally thank all of them, the list would be too long. But over the years, some have stood out as my right hands, my left hands, and my pillars of strength. Medicine is a team sport, especially when it involves treating sick children. Having fantastic colleagues makes it that much more satisfying and successful. Over the years, we have laughed together, cried together, and really come together, especially in tough situations. The amazing pediatric anesthesiologists: Ihab Ayad, Judith Brill, John Chalabi, Mohammed Iravani, Mary Keyes, Swati Patel, Wendy Ren, Joel Stockman, and Sam Wald at UCLA have made coming to work a pleasure. I feel safe when they are with me, as do my patients. They have the challenging task of establishing a relationship with a child who's about to undergo surgery, explaining risks while at the same time comforting their parents, and making a safe plan for anesthesia in a matter of minutes. They do this with incredible ease — bringing smiles to kids' faces, calming concerned parents, and providing excellent care seamlessly. My operating room and clinic days could not happen without top-notch nursing teams — Nancy Villegas, Diane Sennott, Erik Phelps,

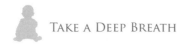

Lolita Nykiel, and David Takenoshita, to name a few, are indispensible. I am also privileged to work with fantastic pediatricians and specialists. Sherin and Uday Devaskar, Rick Harrison, Mariam Ischander, Paul Krogstad, Dan Levi, Andy Madikians, Gary Rachelefsky, Pornchai Tirakitsoontorn, Fernando Vinuela, Irwin Weiss, and Heide Woo, among others, are the reasons why many critically ill children who we treat can eventually thrive at home, out of the hospital. I am also grateful to my own children's pediatrician, Lisa Stern, who simultaneously enables me to be a parent, nervous mom, and colleague.

This book has been many years in the making, and I could not have begun it, dug into it, or completed it without the support and wisdom of Amy Rennert. Amy is not only an amazing and talented literary agent — she has been a friend and role model since we were kids having grown up just five houses from one another. Over the years, we have taken varied turns in our lives and careers, but have both circuitously migrated west, and have found that our paths have merged in our shared love of the written word. She has helped me navigate this uncharted territory of book writing, and to her I am indebted for seeing it through. I am also grateful to Robyn Russell at the Amy Rennert Agency for her help and support and to Louise Kollenbaum for her aesthetic eye.

I wish to thank a great team at World Scientific Publishers for making this book happen. I especially thank for my editor, Sonal Khetarpal, as well as Jimmy Low and Yubing Zhai. Their professionalism and vision have added so much to this finished product.

Amy Sommer — connoisseur, agent to everything, reader, writer, motivator, connector, and friend has been a savior to me. She seems to have an answer to any question, has her finger on many pulses (you'd think she was in the medical field), and has given me entrée to a new world of tweets, sites, virtual reality, good suits, and good hair. Susan Sheu — writer, reader, performer, friend, and voice of calm and reason to me, has made countless suggestions to both strengthen and soften the message of this book. Joanna Moore — neighbor, friend, and a better runner than I can ever dream to be, has also made great recommendations to help make this book as good as it could be. Susanne Resnick has been with me through many iterations of book ideas and titles, from the earliest musings of a breathing book.

My own family has been my biggest and brightest support through this and so many other processes in my life. My parents, Dee and Stan, have given me the unconditional love and encouragement every child should have. My brother, Adam, has always been a superhero to me — he balances more endeavors than ten people could, and actually has a good time doing it. My extended family — Pamela, Benjamin, Zara, Vivi, Marty, Nicole Ross, Cammy, and Will give joy to us and our children, and we are blessed to have them. And of course the day-to-day — home from work, dinners, baths, homework, lessons, plays, shows, story times, bedtimes — are what keeps me going. My husband, Elliot Abemayor (or "Elliot Shapiro" as he jokes when we run into my patients) is a talented and superb head and neck surgeon — treating the most complex, high-risk cancer patients on a daily basis. He comes home to two young children, a tired wife, and Cheerios® and Legos® on the floor after a long day in surgery — but that moment of walking through the door is always his 'rose of the day'. He has been a reader for me, a kind critic, and a supreme inspiration, while at the same time, making sure that I take a break from *Take a Deep Breath* every now and then. Alessandra and Charles, the lights of our lives, truly our breaths of fresh air, never cease to amaze us. Your children will never cease to amaze you, either.

INTRODUCTION

Justin was five months old when I met him. He was a beautiful boy, the second son to a family of privilege in every way — they lived in a remote part of an island paradise, they were loving, had support from extended family and friends, and had already enjoyed the development of their first born son from infant to playful toddler. But something was not right with Justin. Unlike his brother, he, and, in turn, his mother, could not sleep for more than 20 minutes at a time before he would wake up gasping for air. His mother held him continually, finding that he was more comfortable upright on her chest. She would feed him as much as he could tolerate, though with each feed he again became exhausted. Awake or asleep, he used all of his energy to breathe. Justin's parents contacted me, and described what had been going on for the past five months. They sent me a video clip: A beautiful boy indeed — fair-haired, angelic, sitting in his bouncy chair, trying to smile for his dad's camera as his mom cooed to him. He wore a trendy baby t-shirt with a picture of a rock star, barely recognizable because of the folds in the shirt, two sizes too big for this little person. Justin was thin. No, Justin was emaciated. He was using all of his strength — all of his muscles — in his neck, chest, and tummy, to breathe. With each breath, I could hear a heart-wrenching squeak.

When they arrived in Los Angeles, I expected to see a disheveled, panicked mom at her wit's end. Instead, she was lovely, so put together, so accepting of Justin's state of being, and so devoted to his every breath. We would all wish to look so great and be so nice on a full night's sleep, let alone 20 minutes at a clip. And Justin was just as he was in the movie — charming, exhausted, and skinny.

Luckily, it turned out that he had a relatively common problem of the voice box which can cause mild to severe breathing problems in babies. In his case, he had one

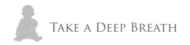

of the most severe cases I've ever seen. The next day, he had a tiny surgery on his tiny airway. That night, next to the big hospital bed dwarfing this little boy, his mother didn't sleep a wink as she watched Justin sleep all night, silently.

While there is nothing more frightening than the feeling of struggling to breathe, watching your child have breathing problems is magnitudes more terrifying. In infancy, you may hover over your newborn's bassinet, 'willing' every breath, wondering if your child will remain peacefully breathing if you were to walk away. Why does my baby stop breathing for several seconds at a time while he sleeps? Why does my baby seem to have trouble breathing and make a snorting sound during feeding? Is this normal? Should I worry? Why does her breathing worsen when sleeping on her back than on her tummy, even though my doctor recommended that she sleeps on her back? Sometimes that little triangle at the bottom of her neck pulls in when she breathes. Will a humidifier help, or make things worse? Do I need to buy an air purifier for the baby's room? Do my walls have lead paint from prior paint jobs? HELP! These and other questions often perplex the most health-savvy of parents.

Your concerns about your child's breathing don't end after the first year. In toddler and preschool years, you may wonder, is my son wheezing because he has asthma, or is that just another one of his colds? Is the snoring and nighttime cough I hear from my daughter common among all two-year-olds? Sometimes my son snores so loudly, he sounds like an old man. Then he seems to hold his breath and take a big gasp before starting to snore again. He seems a little crankier than usual in the morning. Is this just part of the 'terrible two' phase, or am I missing something? Is it okay if my child always breathes with his mouth open? Why is her nose always stuffed, but when she blows it, nothing comes out? Is she too young to see an allergist? And what in the world could be growing in her carpet?

When your child enters daycare or preschool, contagious respiratory illnesses become rampant, and issues of snoring and wheezing may begin to impact his ability to concentrate, focus, and learn. What may have seemed to be just 'cute', stuffy-nosed breathing or adorable snoring of a two-year-old may become more concerning when these peculiar noises begin to take their toll. You may also see that some respiratory conditions can be more debilitating on a day-to-day basis. Why does my five-year-old still get so many colds? I thought those were a problem of babies! Why do my daughter's colds last so long? How do I know if she's having more than a cold, or even sinusitis? She always has dark circles under her eyes. Is she sleep-deprived, allergic, or both? Do I need to bring her to the pediatrician with each of these prolonged colds, and how long is too long?

In *Take a Deep Breath*, I will clearly explain all of those puzzling and oftentimes concerning breathing patterns our children have throughout their development. From the uppermost part of the breathing apparatus, the nose, to the lowermost part, the lungs, I will explain which breathing problems are truly worrisome, and which are actually a normal part of your child's growth. I'll tease out the truth from the hype regarding 'clean', 'green' home environments, and give you suggestions on what you can do to protect your child from breathing in harmful chemicals and allergens. I'll also describe what really happens to your child when she breathes the air both inside and out of your home. In *Take a Deep Breath*, I will enable you to do just that, take a deep breath, and get a better, clearer understanding about what's going on when your children breathe in and out.

The air quality of your home is a key factor in keeping your child's breathing healthy. Young children spend the majority of their day at home, with many of these hours spent sleeping. You will get the nitty gritty on how and what you can do to keep the air your young one breathes as clean and safe as possible, but avoid the unnecessary gimmicks that we all hear about, but are actually of no value at all. You will find out the best, easiest technique to clean a newborn's nasal passage, the first thing to do if a child chokes on food, the #1 and #2 most important home treatments for a baby with croup, and how to hold a nebulizer mask on a busy toddler.

Respiratory problems in children are now also being recognized as *acquired* from the environment, and not just due to bad genes or bad luck. The press is filled with scares and hypes about in-home and outdoor pollutants, 'poisoning' our children. I will clearly lay out the truth from the scams about allergens, environmental pollutants, in-home chemicals, and global warming as they may impact your child's breathing. Beyond simply recommending that you should support the EPA and go 'green', I will provide reasonable, usable guidelines to 'clear the air' for your children.

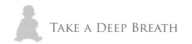

I've arranged the book by age-based sections, and each section will include location-based and problem-based chapters. In each chapter, I will also provide you with 'To-Do' lists, offering successful preventions and treatments that can easily be done at home. Each 'To-Do' list will give pointers and techniques on what can be done, and, more importantly, *how* it can be done at home, to ease breathing problems.

While I break things down by age range and body parts, I realize that many children of course have multiple levels of problem areas contributing to their body's breathing troubles. A 'Big Picture', a 'Don't Worry' and a 'Worry' section at the end of each chapter will be great to use as quick references, as they will highlight and remind you of what you may have forgotten to check for when your baby is sick.

Take a Deep Breath does not take the place of a healthcare professional's evaluation, recommendations, or treatment of your child's breathing issues. But I will provide you with the latest information on what is really going on with your child's breathing, from the inside as well as from the outside. I will incorporate my experience of over 15 years of treating tens of thousands of children with breathing issues, with the latest, most salient information from the medical literature. I will also include the most up-to-date recommendations from prominent pediatric societies such as the American Academy of Pediatrics and the American Society of Pediatric Otolaryngology, as well as valuable facts from reputable non-medical sources in the print and web-based literature. While this is not a medical book, I do use some medical terminology, which will be in **bold**. The meaning and significance of these words will be explained in both the text itself as well as in the Appendix.

I have been writing this book in my head for years, treating countless children and families who feel a bit lost in what is happening with their child's breathing. I hope to enlighten many, provide some insight and resources for help, and empower both adults and children to get a handle on that 'in and out' silent breathing that we take for granted until a problem arises. So sit back, relax, and take a deep breath.

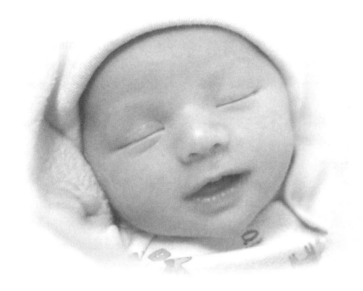

NEWBORN TO
THREE MONTHS

This age group is often the most frightening
for parents. Newborns are so small, fragile,
and vulnerable. Seemingly minor variations
in breathing patterns are oftentimes call for alarm.

1

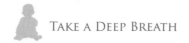

I n these chapters, I will explain the normal variations in newborn breathing patterns, and describe clearly what should and should not be happening to your baby's breathing. I will tease out the truth from the exaggerations about how to truly 'clear the air' for your newborn's home, and what is safe as far as outdoor exposure, public places, and, eventually, travel environments. As with all of the sections, I will take you from the nose to the lungs, explaining why newborns must breathe through their nose, how to keep their noses clean and open, and why eating and breathing are so closely linked, especially in young infants. This section will also explain controversies in sleep positioning, and why it is so important to have your baby sleep on his back until he's able to turn himself over on his own. I will also point out the differences between a simple cold and something more serious such as bronchitis or pneumonia. When dealing with a sick newborn, it's often times hard for both new and experienced parents to decide whether to make that midnight phone call to the pediatrician, go back to sleep, go to the emergency room, or call 911. This section will give you guidelines to help you make those difficult decisions. I will also discuss Sudden Infant Death Syndrome (SIDS), explain its possible causes and risk factors, and more importantly, describe ways that will minimize your baby's risk of experiencing this devastating event.

Chapter One

Nose-Breathing a Must!

All parents-to-be look forward to hearing their newborn's first cry, mouth wide open. But did you know that your baby cannot breathe through his mouth, EXCEPT when crying? That's right. Newborns MUST breathe through their nose, if they want to breathe at all. They are what we call **obligate nasal breathers**. They have not yet developed the complex reflex that tells them to open their mouth to breathe if their nose is blocked. When you or an older child has a stuffy nose, you may sound a little funny, but you simply breathe through your mouth until your nose gets clear. Until approximately age four months, infants cannot do this. The only way by which they can breathe through their mouth is by crying.

If your baby has a severe nasal blockage, doctors and nurses usually discover this in the delivery room. They will see a baby with a normal cry who cannot breathe when not crying. The delivery room staff will then place small plastic **suction catheters** in each nasal passage of your newborn baby. These catheters look like long, clear, floppy cocktail straws and serve two purposes: (1) they suction and remove any fluids the baby may have retained while being in a water-filled environment for nine months; and (2) they determine whether or not a baby has open nasal air passages for breathing. Even if a baby has only one open nasal passage, he will be able to breathe through that one nostril, usually without requiring any emergency treatment. Severe complete nasal airway blockage (**choanal atresia**), is a rare occurrence (approximately 1 in 4000 births). If your baby does have this, it can be treated with a small surgery, usually in the first few weeks of his birth.

In this chapter, I will give you helpful hints on how to handle that stuffy newborn, explain what's inside your baby's nose and how that tiny nose works, and let you know why it's so important.

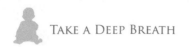

***Ever since we've brought our baby home, she makes funny snorting
noises, especially when she feeds.***

Since newborns are **obligate nasal breathers** (they HAVE to breathe through their
nose), any nasal blockage will be quite noisy, and may even make the baby uncomfortable. The nasal passages in newborns are tiny, only about 2–3 millimeters (about
one tenth of one inch) on each side, so it takes very little change in that small space
to cause big symptoms. Think of your baby's nose as a tiny greenhouse: it needs
moisture, warmth, air filtration, ventilation, and greenery. The mucous lining of the
nose provides the moisture. This lining has tiny glands that supply the wet, slippery
mucus that keeps the nose from becoming a crusted desert, and allows air to flow
freely. The warmth is provided by body temperature and the small dark space in the
nasal cavity. The filtering is accomplished by both tiny nose hairs and by the slippery
mucus (the greenery), so that dust and dirt are not breathed directly into the lungs.
They catch and collect particles, filtering them out from the air your baby breathes.
Ventilation is provided by the open nasal passage that connects the outside world
to the back of the nose.

   Since the nasal passages in babies are so small, their work of producing mucus
and catching dust may cause swelling of the nasal tissues. This common problem
is called **neonatal rhinitis**. This is the medical term for 'stuffy nose of the newborn',
and most babies gradually grow out of this in the first one to two months of life.
It may be due to a little congestion from their new air- and dust-filled environment, or from a slight, temporary narrowing in the nasal passages. Since they need
to breathe through their noses, the snorting and grunting can be quite disconcerting. You may notice that these noises escalate during feeding times. The sucking
motion, whether by breastfeeding or bottle feeding, requires a lot of energy, and
the motion of sucking pulls the baby's tongue up towards the soft part of the roof
of the mouth (**soft palate**). In the newborn, the roof of the mouth is so close to
the back of the nose, this action may actually block the nose even more. If the
nose is not wide open for breathing, your baby may not be able to coordinate such
complex muscle activities of sucking, eating, and breathing. Your baby with a stuffy
nose may take longer to finish a feed, and may take frequent rest breaks to finish.
Even a little dried mucus can cause certain nasal breathing problems, especially
during feeding.

In most cases, this nasal congestion during feeding is easily remedied by using **nasal saline** drops before feedings. There is no dangerous chemical or medication in saline, and nasal saline can be purchased over-the-counter at most drugstores or supermarkets. It contains sterilized water and salt, mixed to a solution that is similar to the salt and water content of the lining of the nose. To use the drops, hold your baby's head upright, so that he won't feel like saline is going right to his throat. Place the nozzle in one side of the baby's nose, and gently squeeze the bottle a few times. Repeat on the other side. Most of the saline will drip back out, but some of it will go where it is needed. Most babies do not like the saline drops being used, but believe it or not, most get used to it and it becomes easier for everybody after several tries. The nasal passages are not angled 'up' to the top of the nose, but are a straight line back. If you are sitting up and make a line with your hand between your nostril and your ear parallel to the floor, that is the direction of the nasal air passage. Keep that in mind when you use any nasal medications. Aim back, not up.

Does suctioning my baby's nose help with her breathing? How often should I do this?

Doctors often recommend nasal suctioning for newborns, and many hospitals send families home with a newborn suction bulb to remove any nasal mucus. While this is helpful in keeping your baby's nasal passages clear, parents often get a little 'suction happy', and use this too frequently, especially with a stuffy baby. I would discourage this, unless large amounts of mucus are visible. Frequent suctioning puts a lot of pressure on the delicate nasal tissues, and can actually lead to more swelling and congestion. So, if your baby is stuffy but not dripping with mucus, minimize suctioning and maximize saline. There is no such thing as using saline drops 'too often'. It is not absorbed into your baby's body, your baby cannot become dependent on it, and it does not cause swelling.

If you have a stuffy nosed baby, a cool mist humidifier also helps to cut down on dryness, crusting, and nasal airway swelling. Cool-mist humidifiers are preferable to warm-mist, as the cool ones tend to breed less bacteria and mold in the water basin. But even if you use a cool-mist humidifier, make sure you clean it regularly. Each brand usually comes with detailed cleaning instructions to minimize contamination.

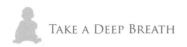
What if I've tried saline, suctioning, and humidifiers, but my baby is still stuffy?

Rarely, babies will have a more severe case of **neonatal rhinitis**, where despite best efforts of saline, minimal suctioning, and humidification, your baby is still uncomfortably stuffy all of the time. This is usually most noticeable during feeding and sleeping. A baby who is having trouble with feedings because of nasal stuffiness, and has difficulty with breathing all the time (chronic snorting, inability to sleep due to snoring or breathing trouble), has more nasal stuffiness than most other newborns. You may notice that the triangle-shaped notch in the lower neck, just above the chest, pulls inward with each breath. This is called a **retraction**. Your pediatrician needs to know about this, as this is a sign that your baby is using extra muscles for breathing, and it may indicate that your baby is struggling. Babies with nasal stuffiness and breathing difficulties are often evaluated by an ear, nose, and throat specialist. These specialists can examine the entire nasal passage, from the front to the back, with a tiny telescope, to make sure that there is nothing blocking the air passages. These determinations can be made in an office visit, and are quick. A tiny drop of local anesthetic is placed in the baby's nose, and the whole examination can take less than a minute. If all that is found is stuffiness, a short course of **steroid** nose drops may be prescribed, or the doctor may simply recommend watchful waiting. Steroids are strong anti-inflammatory medications, but if used as local drops, there is no concern about significant absorption into the bloodstream. If there is a physical blockage in the nose, your doctor may recommend a type of X-ray called a CT (**computed tomography**) scan of the nose, to look for cysts, tumors, or bony overgrowths in the nose. This degree of nasal blockage is quite rare (less than one percent of babies), and the need for these scans is just as rare.

Our six-week old baby has caught her first cold. She is so uncomfortable — she can't eat well, sleep well, or get comfortable in any position. What can we do?

Whether or not your newborn baby has exposure to other children, she is likely to get at least one cold before the age of three months, especially if her birthday is in the fall or winter. Minor colds in young infants affect primarily their noses, and, since they are **obligate nasal breathers**, this is quite distressing. These are times when even babies with completely normal nasal passages will benefit from nasal saline drops or spray, room humidification, and even gentle suctioning if there is a lot of mucus involved. **Oxymetazoline (Afrin[R])** drops, which can be purchased over the counter at most pharmacies, are often safe to use in infants if mixed half and half with saline in the bottle (you can do this yourself at home). It is a topical **decongestant** that will shrink some of the swollen tissue which lines that delicate nasal passage, and will allow your baby to breathe more comfortably. It will not make her cold go away any faster, but it may alleviate some of those nights of snorting and crying. While most physicians are comfortable using this medication in young infants, *you should check with your doctor* to see if this is safe for your baby. If your doctor says it is safe for your baby, then you can use it for up to two days, two times per day. Squirt twice into each nostril with the bottle upright. (Remember 2-2-2: 2 sprays, 2 times per day, for 2 days). If you prefer the drop method, you can turn the bottle upside down and use a few drops on each side, but stick with the 2-2-2 rule. Using oxymetazoline for more than two to three days can cause what's called a **rebound response**, whereby longer term use will actually have the reverse effect, and your baby's nose (or yours, if you are using it) will become more and more swollen and congested over time.

If your baby has simply a stuffy and/or runny nose with no fever, lethargy, or inability to feed, either by breast or bottle, it is likely the first of many minor colds to come. However, any stuffy or runny nose in an infant in the presence of fever greater than 100 degrees Fahrenheit, decreased energy, or inability to feed warrants a call to your doctor right away. The issue of fever raises an important point. Make sure that you have at least one digital thermometer before you bring your baby home from the hospital. Babies are extremely poor at temperature regulation, so you cannot rely on kissing their forehead or guessing how warm their body temperature is. This is one of many instances where technology is your friend. Any digital thermometer should work just fine. It does not need to be the fanciest

RULE OF TWO'S FOR OXYMETAZOLINE SPRAY:

TWO DROPS
TWO TIMES PER DAY
TWO DAYS

one with the bells and whistles. Most standard digital thermometers sold in drug-stores work just fine. In an infant, you can check body temperature in one of several ways: rectal temperature: gently place the tip into your baby's bottom. While this is the most uncomfortable, it is the quickest and most accurate method of measuring body temperature. Make sure that this particular thermometer is labeled as your rectal one — even if it's washed, you wouldn't want to use it for an oral temperature on even the closest of family members. You can also measure your baby's temperature by placing the tip of the thermometer in her armpit, and then holding her arm down so that the thermometer is snug in that skin fold until the thermometer beeps. This is slightly less accurate than a rectal temperature, and tends to 'under' record the temperature by about one degree Fahrenheit, but does give a pretty close measure of temperature, especially if there is a high fever. Other options are temperature stickers — which need to be placed on your baby's forehead for several minutes. They are easy to use, and disposable, but may be hard to read accurately. Ear thermometers are hand-held gadgets whose small tip is placed into your baby's ear canal. These are usually quite easy to use, give quick answers, are easy to read, and are accurate. They also come with disposable tips, which lessens concern for spreading germs when the family thermometer gets passed around.

Our baby seems to have thick, rubber cement-like mucus coming out of one side of her nose. What could this be?

While infants are **obligate nasal breathers**, they only *need* one side of their nose to do this. If a baby has complete blockage of one nasal passage, the natural flow of mucus will not be there, and the mucus that is produced will remain in the nasal passage and become quite thick. Their 'greenhouse' has no ventilation. This will not clear with saline drops, and will require frequent suctioning. Most babies with this one-sided blockage will not have significant breathing trouble, but they may require a specialist to evaluate them. Possible reasons that a baby may have rubber cement-like mucus include complete blockage of one side of the nose, either at the very front part or at the very back part, formation of cysts, which are fluid-filled sacs that may develop before or soon after birth, or growths of solid tissue, which may also form either before or after birth.

Our baby had a very traumatic vaginal delivery, and it seems as if his nose was pushed to one side and it looks crooked. The left side of his nose looks blocked. Is he headed for plastic surgery? Did he break his nose?

Very rarely, during vaginal delivery, the baby's nose can get compressed against the back part of the mom's **pelvic bone** during delivery. Newborn nasal bones are very soft and pliable, so a nasal fracture (where the bone is actually broken) is quite unusual. However, it is possible to have a crooked nose at birth. If it is barely visible, and seems to be better/straighter in two or three days after birth, chances are it was just some nasal swelling that will resolve in a matter of a week or so. If it is visibly very obvious, you may also see that the **nasal septum** (the cartilage that separates the right side of the nose from the left side) is deviated. This may cause breathing problems. If there is a severe nasal deformity, usually seen as either the tip of the nose curving off to one side, or as one side of the nose blocked by the septum, then an ear, nose, and throat specialist should evaluate your baby. They may be able to gently push these pliable tissues (even bone) back into place in the first week of his life. It is surprisingly not too uncomfortable, and can usually be done in the doctor's office or before leaving the hospital after birth.

THE BIG PICTURE

While newborns rely on those tiny nasal air passages, and the snorting, grunting noises they make when there is some blockage of airflow may *sound* terrible, what is more important is how your baby is *doing* overall. The best way to assess whether a baby is okay is whether they are *thriving*. And a great way to determine whether or not you have a thriving baby is weight gain. Babies should gain anywhere from roughly ½ to one ounce per day (one to two pounds per month), after the initial ½ to ¾ pound weight loss in the first week of life. If a baby is gaining weight appropriately, chances are she is thriving, and a stuffy nose is not getting in her way. On the other hand, if your baby is using so much energy to breathe while working around that stuffy nose, her calorie expenditure may lead to poor weight gain. Pediatricians usually monitor newborns quite closely if there is a breathing issue, and weight gain is a big factor in determining whether the baby is okay or not, and whether or not she is in need of further evaluation or treatment.

DON'T WORRY

If your baby makes snorting noises, but is sleeping comfortably, and is eating and gaining weight, any nasal stuffiness will likely be short-lived and easily treated with over-the-counter saline nose drops, a room humidifier, and time.

WORRY

If your baby is snorting, but at the same time has to frequently struggle to breathe (**retractions** — you will see that triangle in the lower neck pull in, the stomach muscles and his chest muscles tightening and pulling inwards between each rib), there is a problem that needs to be addressed by your doctor right away. If you notice that your baby's nostrils are flaring, that is also a sign that she is struggling. If your baby tires with each feed because of breathing troubles, this may also indicate a problem. ANY time your baby has an episode of turning blue in the lips or face (**cyanosis**), this is a problem, and you need to seek medical attention immediately.

TO-DO LIST: NOSE-BREATHING A MUST!

1. Remember, any life-threatening nasal blockage is usually discovered in the delivery room or soon after, and your doctor will be able to evaluate and manage these problems right after birth.

2. Nose-breathing is what newborns rely on to get air into their lungs.

3. Nasal saline (over-the-counter, any brand) should be on hand at your changing table, as well as in your diaper bag.

4. You can never use saline too often.

5. Nasal saline is oftentimes more effective than nasal suctioning.

6. When using nasal saline, hold your baby's head upright. Put the nozzle of the spray bottle in a nostril, and then give a few good squirts, in a backward direction

(not upward). Most of the saline will drip out, but her nose will be remarkably irrigated. Repeat on the other side.

7. If your baby prefers lying on his back, turn the saline bottle upside down and gently drip a few drops into each nostril. He may cough a little, but it wont hurt him.

8. If your baby is very congested with a cold, check with your doctor about using **oxymetazoline** spray/drops to relieve severe stuffiness. Apply as you would nasal saline, but use this medication no more than two times per day for no more than two days at a time (The 2-2-2 Rule).

9. Remember the moisture of the "greenhouse" you need to maintain: a humidifier, cool mist is best, especially during air conditioner or dry heat use.

10. To check if your baby is breathing through her nose, hold the corner of a tissue just outside the nostril. If the tissue moves back and forth, there is air going in and out.

11. If one side of your baby's nose always has thick mucus (like rubber cement), and the other side does not, there may be a structural problem that needs to be addressed by your doctor. Such problems are a nuisance, but almost never an emergency.

Source for Nose-Breathing in Newborns:
http://pediatric-ent.com/learning/problems/nasal_obstruction.htm

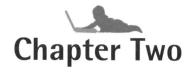

Chapter Two

Throaty Gurgles: The Low-Down on the Lazy Voice Box

Babies make the strangest noises, either while eating, sleeping, or just 'being'. Where are these sounds coming from, and should you be concerned? In this chapter, you will learn that your baby's **voice box** and upper **esophagus** (swallowing food tube) are just at the back of his tongue. Understanding that these structures are within the space of a few fractions of an inch in a newborn will help you make sense of all of these sounds. If you think about it, there is so much coordination and work that needs to be done in such a small space. In a few fractions of an inch, your tiny baby needs to get air into one hole, and food into another, often simultaneously. This coordination has to occur quickly, as babies breathe from 24 to 38 times per minute. But just like other newborn mammals, they manage to do it. Their reflexes are wired well before leaving the fluid-filled, cozy, warm prenatal environment, entering the cold, aerated world.

Many sounds your baby makes sound like a stuffy nose, and in many cases a stuffy nose it is (see Chapter One). On the other hand, her other breathing structures (voice box, **palate**, and tongue) are so close to the back of her nose, that what sounds like 'nasal' stuffiness may actually be something else. You may notice that his 'nose' becomes stuffy after eating, or when he's upset. But is it really his nose? Maybe not. In this chapter, I will explain those sounds — what you are hearing, why you are hearing it, and tricks of the trade to help your baby.

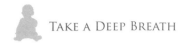

Our baby sometimes seems like she's choking, with little brief gasps of air. It seems as if there's something stuck for a few seconds, and then she seems fine.

Newborns have a lot to coordinate in a very small space. They need air to pass through their air passage, and food to pass through their swallow passage. This can sometimes cause a bit of air/food traffic jam.

The structures of the air passage that sit right above the windpipe are part of the **larynx**, which is another name for voice box. The **epiglottis** sits at the top part of the larynx and is a leaf-like flap of tissue that protects the windpipe from foreign objects and does not let anything except air from getting in. It is made of cartilage, similar in consistency to the cartilage of your ear or windpipe (**trachea**). Sometimes in newborns, the epiglottis is a bit floppy, and, instead of stiff cartilage, it is like soft skin. When your baby breathes in, her epiglottis should open up like blooming flower. However, if her epiglottis is floppy, it will close on itself like a tightening fist. The 'choking' noise you hear is that floppy epiglottis closing on itself. Sometimes you can hear a clicking sound with each breath, as your baby is trying to pull air in through a floppy, closing space.

A baby with a floppy epiglottis has what is known as **laryngomalacia**. Laryngomalacia means that the protective cartilage above the windpipe is still soft, and has not yet developed into a firmer consistency. In babies with laryngomalacia, the voice box is not quite doing its job correctly, making it seem somewhat 'lazy'. However, it is usually just a matter of time before this 'laziness' will go away on its own. Laryngomalacia is commonly seen in premature babies, but full-term babies often have this as well. It may be mild, where you occasionally hear the 'clicking' noises, more often when your baby is excited, being fed, just finishing a feed, or crying. It may be moderate, where you hear the noise more often, even when they seem to be resting comfortably. Or it may be severe, where the noise is very loud, you hear it all the time, and your baby has **retractions**, where you see the muscles of the lower neck, between the ribs, or the stomach pulling in with each breath. The terms, 'mild', 'moderate' and 'severe' refer to the degree of noise and symptoms that your baby has, as well as to the degree of 'floppiness' of the epiglottis. The floppier the epiglottis, the more severe the laryngomalacia. It is not known why some babies have mild laryngomalacia, some have moderate, and some have severe. They are all on the spectrum of the same diagnosis, although the time course and treatment varies based on these degrees.

If your baby is experiencing any of these noises, your pediatrician will most likely refer you to an ear, nose, and throat doctor. The ear, nose, and throat doctor will look at your baby's throat with a tiny camera during an office visit, and will be able to see if laryngomalacia is the reason for the noise.

What if my baby is diagnosed with MILD laryngomalacia?

Mild laryngomalacia is actually quite common. Up to 10% of newborns have some degree of laryngomalacia. In mild laryngomalacia, the tissue of the epiglottis is a little bit floppy, but has some strength which keeps things open (like that blooming flower). In these babies, quiet breathing is more the norm, but they do occasionally have periods of noisy clicking/choking sounds. While the sounds may be quite distressing to you, your baby probably won't seem particularly bothered by this. These babies are happily making noise, more so with excitement, crying, or during or after a feeding. They don't have any retractions, and have no problems breathing during feeding or during sleep. These babies have comfortable, quiet breathing while sleeping on their backs (which is the American Academy of Pediatrics (AAP) recommended position until your baby can turn over on his own).

Mild laryngomalacia is self-limited. The noise is usually noticed soon after birth, or in the first few weeks thereafter. The noise itself may get louder for the first four to six months, and eventually goes away on its own before your baby's first birthday. No particular treatment is needed. You may notice that the noise goes away when your baby is held in the upright position (this is especially helpful during and after feeding), or is sitting in a car seat or in an infant swing. This is because the elevation and extra support of his neck helps to open the air passage.

ABOUT 10% OF BABIES HAVE SOME DEGREE OF LARYNGOMALACIA

Why, you may ask, if the laryngomalacia is so mild, does it get worse (louder) before it gets better? The reason for this is that the tissue grows faster than it firms up. As the epiglottis grows before it firms

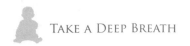
up, it may get temporarily floppier, leading to louder noise, though just temporarily. Another reason for the 'noisier' breathing is that, as your baby grows, he becomes more active. He is more alert, can get more excited, begins to smile, interact, and even move freely. The increased activity increases the rate and force of his breathing, which may bring with it more noise. Because there is a period of 'noisier' breathing in mild cases of laryngomalacia, your doctor may want to check your baby's progress every few months, until the noise goes away completely.

What if my baby is diagnosed with MODERATE laryngomalacia?

Moderate laryngomalacia is also relatively common. These babies have a floppy epiglottis, but you may notice that the noisy breathing is present more often than not. Your baby's breathing may become much noisier during or after feeding, and it may be worse when she is sleeping on her back. DO NOT BE TEMPTED TO PUT YOUR NEWBORN BABY ON HER STOMACH TO SLEEP. Although her breathing may seem better, it is still not recommended to do this. Her breathing can be compromised while sleeping on her stomach, even though it may seem to sound better to you. If your baby is having a lot of trouble breathing while on her back, there are options to help with this. One is to obtain a wedge for the crib or bassinette. This elevates her head, while allowing her to stay on her *back* (remember, "BACK to sleep"). Another option is to have your baby sleep in a swing or a car seat. You may not need to do this all the time, but these create a more 'permanent' elevated position during sleep. You may only need to do this sometimes, or during naps. If you have any questions about sleep positions, check with your doctor.

If your baby has moderate laryngomalacia, you also may notice that the noise becomes pretty loud during or after feeds. The reason for this is that the milk or formula is hitting up against that floppy epiglottis, which may cause your baby to choke or sputter. The epiglottis of a newborn sits at the back of the tongue, and is a direct target for milk. In babies with laryngomalacia, the floppiness of the epiglottis makes it a bit longer and stretched out, making it easier for milk to hit it. If you are breast-feeding, your milk may come out too quickly (especially after the first week or two of breastfeeding), and your baby may have trouble protecting her air passage as the milk hits that epiglottis. Keeping her somewhat upright during feeds may help with this. While it is hard to control your milk flow, you may need to give your baby 'breathing breaks' during a feed, beyond the usual breaks for burping. These 'breathing breaks' allow for her to get her breathing and swallowing coordinated, as well as to cough out any milk that may have hit up against the epiglottis. If your baby is bottle-fed, make sure that you have a 'low-flow' nipple. While it may take longer for a feed, the slowed speed of the milk or formula means that less will hit up against the epiglottis with each swallow, giving your baby more time to get it past that floppy tissue.

Babies with moderate laryngomalacia may also have significant worsening of the noise as they become more active. As with babies who have mild laryngomalacia, the epiglottis may grow faster than it firms up, making the noise much louder and coarser. If your baby still seems comfortable during these noisy periods, there is nothing to be concerned about. However, if you feel that your baby is struggling to breathe during this time, let your doctor know right away. The good news is, that by the end of her third month, her head control begins to kick in, where the neck muscles supporting her head take over. This also helps to keep her breathing passage more vertical and open.

What if my baby was diagnosed with SEVERE laryngomalacia?

A very small percentage of newborns with laryngomalacia are diagnosed with severe laryngomalacia. These babies will have noisy breathing more often, whether they are eating, sleeping, resting, or crying. The noise will be loud, and you will hear it with almost each breath. It may even sound like a quick, little high-pitched shriek or scream each time he breathes in. You may likely be able to hear it from the next room. These babies may have more significant retractions, of either the neck muscles, chest muscles, or abdominal muscles. Sleeping will be more challenging, as proper positioning will be more critical, and feeding will be more difficult, whereby your baby may have more breathing trouble during and after feeds.

THE AMERICAN ACADEMY OF PEDIATRICS RECOMMENDS THAT ALL INFANTS BE PLACED ON THEIR BACKS WHEN BEING PUT DOWN TO SLEEP

Babies with severe laryngomalacia are much more comfortable in the upright position, and it may be an option to have him sleep in a car seat or swing during daytime naps as well as at night. In

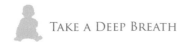

these cases, even a wedge at the crib's head may not be enough to help with breathing. In very young infants, make sure that you have side head supports in the car seat of swing to keep his head centered. Sometimes having your baby sleep almost 'sitting,' temporarily, will get him through a tough phase. Check with your pediatrician to see if this is an option.

Feeding a baby with severe laryngomalacia has many challenges. Very frequent breaks are required for your baby to catch his breath. But if he is getting enough quantity-wise, there is little to be concerned about. If you are bottle-feeding, it is easy to gauge how much he is getting. If you are breastfeeding, you may have to go by your baby's weight gain. This brings up an important point: your baby's most important job at this stage is to gain weight. A newborn with a severe breathing problem may not be able to do this. Some newborns with breathing problems can't get enough volume in, because it's so difficult to eat and breathe at the same time. Some newborns can't gain weight because they are burning calories while breathing, and despite adequate intake, can't gain weight due to all of those extra calories burned. Your doctor may want you to bring your baby in for weekly weight checks, to make sure that things are moving in the right direction. Babies at this stage should gain an average of approximately ½ to 1 ounce per day (one to two pounds per month).

Another concern in babies with severe laryngomalacia is that their breathing difficulties may begin to impact their overall health. Babies with severe laryngomalacia may have prolonged periods of **apnea** (absence of breathing), where they stop breathing for several seconds at a time, despite trying to breathe. In general, newborns have very irregular breathing patterns, and may commonly have periods of apnea WITHOUT making efforts to breathe. This is called **central apnea**, and for the most part, is due to immature breathing reflexes. This is most commonly seen during sleep. However, **obstructive apnea** is an entity where your baby is making efforts to breathe against physical blockage, such as a floppy epiglottis. Babies with severe laryngomalacia commonly have obstructive apneas, either during wake time or sleep time. You may notice that they pull their neck muscles in, tighten up their body, and then take a gasp for air. Babies can usually handle these episodes pretty well. However, apnea can lead to **cyanosis** ('blue' spells). If there is a long enough period of apnea (absence of breathing), lack of oxygen will lead to a blue discoloration of the skin, usually first seen on the lips or under the fingernails. The type of cyanosis associated with apnea or a breathing problem, however, needs to be differentiated from **acral cyanosis**. Acral cyanosis is where you see a blue tinge to the skin of the palms, soles, area around the lips, or even at the tip of their nose. This type of cyanosis ('blueness') is due to the immaturity of an infant's temperature regulation. You may see them breathing comfortably, but occasionally develop that blue tinge around their lips (not their lips themselves), nose, on their hands, or on their feet. A newborn may appear blue around her extremities or lips after coming out of a warm bath. Her temperature regulation is immature, and sometimes it takes extra time for the blood from the lungs to re-distribute, with the extremities filling up last. Either way, EVEN ONE BLUE SPELL MERITS A CALL TO YOUR DOCTOR, especially if you're not sure which type it was.

A small percentage of babies with severe laryngomalacia may need a surgical procedure to help 'open' up their floppy epiglottis. This is reserved for babies who are having either continuous retractions, poor weight gain (or weight loss) due to their breathing problem, or blue spells with apnea. The surgery is performed through their mouth with tiny surgical instruments, with visualization by telescopes and digital camera systems. There are no cuts or stitches on the outside. Babies may have a minimal sore throat afterwards, but most babies are able to feed right after surgery, and their breathing improves either immediately, or within a day or two after surgery. They will usually need to stay in the hospital for a few days afterwards for monitoring, and almost all hospitals let you stay with your baby 24 hours per day after surgery. This procedure does not 'fix' the laryngomalacia, but it does lessen the degree of symptoms, and enables the severity to go away faster.

NEWBORN BABIES SHOULD GAIN ½ TO 1 OUNCE PER DAY, OR 1 TO 2 POUNDS PER MONTH

THE BIG PICTURE

Laryngomalacia (floppy epiglottis) is a surprisingly common problem in newborns. The majority of babies with laryngomalacia will have 'noisy' breathing soon after birth. You and the hospital staff or pediatrician may even notice it before you go home from the hospital. Alternatively, you may not notice it until your baby is several weeks old. If your baby is diagnosed with laryngomalacia (it needs to be done so with a tiny camera); the ear, nose, and throat doctor will tell you whether it is mild, moderate, or severe. These differentiations are made not only based on how things look (a little floppy, quite floppy, incredibly floppy), but on how your baby sounds and how he has been doing. This will also determine what measures you need to do at home as far as is positioning after feeding, during rest, and during sleep is concerned, and how often you need to see your pediatrician and/or specialist. The vast majority of babies with laryngomalacia grow out of it on their own, with minimal treatment. As with any airway problem, laryngomalacia symptoms worsen when your baby gets a respiratory infection. These babies need closer attention by their doctor when they get a cold.

DON'T WORRY

If your baby makes occasional 'clicking' noises, is diagnosed with laryngomalacia, but is comfortable, eating properly, sleeping well, and is happy, don't let these noises bother you. More likely than not, the noises will bother other people more than they bother you or your baby. 'Is your baby ok?' 'Did you know he's making a funny noise?' may be the common questions asked by complete strangers. 'Yes' is enough of an answer to them. Or, 'Yes, but where did you get that ugly hat?'

WORRY

If your baby makes constant and very loud clicking noises, with retractions of the neck or chest, has trouble with feeds because of breathing issues, or has any blue spells, this is a reason to call your doctor right away, or even go to an emergency room, especially if the noise/struggling becomes worse over the course of a few hours or days.

TO-DO LIST: THE LOW-DOWN ON THE LAZY VOICE BOX

1. If your baby has mild, moderate, or severe floppy epiglottis (laryngomalacia), remember that it is a very common condition (seen in up to 10% of newborns), and it will eventually go away.

2. Most babies with laryngomalacia will have their symptoms worsened during or after feeds, while crying, and sometimes when sleeping on their back.

3. Keep your baby as upright as possible during feeding, and keep him in this position for at least twenty minutes after each feed. This will allow for any milk or formula that may have gotten stuck on that floppy epiglottis to be cleared away by your baby's coughing or natural swallowing.

4. Keep your baby as upright as possible during sleep — this may take some trial and error. Options include a wedge to be placed in the bassinett or crib, having your baby sleep in a swing, or having him sleep in an infant's car seat.

5. Laryngomalacia has degrees of severity, but these are not necessarily set in stone. If your baby is diagnosed with mild laryngomalacia, but his breathing becomes more labored, call your doctor right away. You may also notice that 'mild' laryngomalacia becomes 'severe' when your baby gets a cold. In fact, there may just be some temporary congestion around the epiglottis. Either way, when in doubt, let your doctor check it out.

Source for the Lazy Voice Box (Laryngomalacia):
http://pediatric-ent.com/learning/problems/breathing_difficulties.htm

Chapter Three

Newborn Breathing Issues Related to Feeding

The breathing and swallowing passages are so close to each other, especially in newborns. This is one of the reasons why feeding problems can lead to breathing problems, and vice versa. Not only is the back of the voice box attached to the front of the swallowing passage, but the voice box in a newborn sits so high up in the throat, that it is pretty much at the back part of the tongue. Food (or in this case, formula or breast milk) has to get past the tongue, jump over the voice box, and land right in the **esophagus** (swallowing passage) without a hitch. Not always an easy task. More and more babies are now being diagnosed with **gastroesophageal reflux disease (GERD)**, which in the past was considered to be a disorder reserved for overweight adults who ate too much spicy food. It is now known that, due to immature muscles in the throat and esophagus, all babies have some degree of gastroesophageal reflux (GER), and some have true gastroesophageal reflux DISEASE (GERD).

My baby spits up some formula every time I burp her. Is this normal? Is she getting in enough food?
Most babies, especially newborns, spit up some of their feeds, even each time they are burped. Sometimes, it may seem like you are chasing your tail, and that everything going in is coming right out. While sometimes it seems like a lot of the feed is coming out, it is usually mixed with the fluid that the stomach itself produces. But how do you know? Well, there are three possibilities if your baby spits up often: (1) your baby is getting enough in, and is just spitting up the excess; (2) your baby is getting TOO

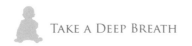

much in, and the overflow is just coming out, like a topped-off gas tank; (3) your baby is getting the right amount, but has a degree of gastroesophageal reflux disease (GERD). In general, babies are excellent self-regulators. If they are satiated after a feed, they will either fall asleep or rest comfortably when it's done, even if they had spit some of it out. If they are overfed, they will let you know by spitting the excess out. If they are unable to keep enough in because of GERD, they will not be 'satisfied' after feeds (a satisfied, fed newborn is usually a sleeping one), and they may require being fed more frequently. Babies with GERD are oftentimes classically described as 'colicky', although this is not always the case. They may not have the arching, wailing misery we hear about (or may be experiencing as you read this) with colic. GERD is not necessarily painful or uncomfortable, but may need to be treated nonetheless.

How do I know if my baby has normal spit-up, overfeeding, or GERD?

All babies have some degree of reflux, which is defined as the backward flow of the stomach's contents to the esophagus and/or throat. Their swallowing muscles are immature, and the **sphincters** (the tighter bands of muscle tissue that prevent the contents from coming up) are also immature. We have a sphincter at the top of our esophagus, separating our esophagus from our mouth, and at the bottom of our esophagus, separating our esophagus from our stomachs. When one or both of these sphincters are 'weak', or in the case of newborns 'immature,' reflux will occur.

Babies with normal spit-up after feeds are usually comfortable during and after feeding. But the best way to determine if your baby has a 'normal' amount of spit-up is by weighing him. Usually pediatricians will weigh newborns every one to three weeks in the first three months, so adequate weight-gain with frequent spit-up is usually not a strong indicator of reflux.

Overfed babies may not spit up, but will literally 'pour' out the feed as it's being completed. The amount is often hard to gauge if your baby is breastfed, but bottle amounts are easier to calculate. Newborns take between two and six ounces in each feed, with these numbers increasing with the baby's age. If you are feeding your baby on the higher end, and the milk or formula just flows right back out of her mouth towards the end of the feed, it may be from over-feeding. Try a smaller amount at a time. If the 'overflow' subsides, after you reduce the amount, it may be an issue of volume overload, not reflux.

GERD may lead to frequent spit-ups or projectile vomiting. Vomiting is considered to be 'projectile' when the vomited material seems to fly across the room, not just pour out of the baby's mouth. Some babies may have pain and irritability, similar to colic, but some may just have frequent spitting up or vomiting, without discomfort. If there is a question of GERD for your baby (usually with a story for high-volume or frequent spit-up, possibly with colicky pain, with neck arching or tummy discomfort during feed), your doctor may want to look into this further. Some pediatricians will recommend testing of your baby's swallowing capacity, either with a **barium swallow study**, where a specialist (radiologist and possibly a speech/swallow specialist) takes X-rays while your baby drinks some white chalky liquid, or a **pH probe**, where a tiny tube is placed from your baby's nose to her stomach, and is left there for several hours, or up to one full day. The pH (a measure of acidity) is recorded from the esophagus to see if stomach acid is creeping up in the wrong direction (the acid content of the esophagus should not be as high as the acid content of the stomach. If this is found, it is a sign of GERD). However, if your baby has a clear history of GERD symptoms, your doctor may give you some recommendations without doing any tests. If your baby improves with these recommendations, no tests may be needed. GERD may be treated by you at home, by giving your baby more frequent, shorter (or lower volume) feeds, and keeping your baby upright for at least 20–30 minutes after each feed. The latter will allow for gravity to keep the milk or formula moving in the right direction, especially if the muscles and sphincters are not doing their jobs. I know it's easy for me to recommend staying up with your baby for an extra 20 minutes, especially after that 3 a.m. feed, when all you want to do is put your baby back to sleep, but those extra few minutes really make a difference. A few extra waking minutes after a feed may give you and your baby a longer sleep period afterwards if their tummy is more settled. If you can't do 20–30 minutes, try for 15 minutes. It really does help. There are several 'anti-reflux' medications that are safe for newborns if non-medical measures are not successful. Very rarely, if the medicine is not helping enough, babies with severe GERD can undergo a surgical procedure to prevent the stomach contents from coming up into the esophagus. This is done as a last resort, but it has an extremely high success rate.

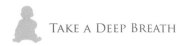

So what does GERD have to do with breathing?

GER and GERD can cause breathing problems in newborns. When the backflow of stomach contents goes up the esophagus, past the upper sphincter, the acidic contents go into the throat and even high up to the back of the nose. These delicate tissues are very sensitive to the acidic stomach contents. As I mentioned, there is a very small distance between the top of the swallowing tube and the back of the throat in newborns, so this age group is the most sensitive to have reflux associated with breathing problems. Newborns with reflux may have coughing, noisy breathing, blue spells, or choking episodes during or right after a feed. But they may or may not have the classic 'spitting-up' we think of with reflux. Evaluation by your doctor is similar to evaluation for GERD in general — possibly some X-ray testing (barium swallow) or acid monitoring (pH probe), but very often the story you give and the exam of your baby (it's especially helpful for your pediatrician to watch your baby during and after a feed) can give an answer. Treating breathing problems caused by reflux is similar to treating reflux in general — more frequent, smaller feeds, keeping your baby upright for at least 20–30 minutes after each feed, and possibly use of medication if the changes in the way the baby is fed do not help.

Babies with breathing problems due to reflux may sound like babies with **laryngomalacia** (see Chapter Two). Their breathing will be noisy, and it will worsen when they are on their backs, after a feed, and when upset. The reason for this is that reflux and laryngomalacia affect the same area in the throat — the **larynx**, or the voice box.

Many babies will actually have both laryngomalacia and GERD. This is because both entities are due to the immaturity of the structures — immature cartilage causes laryngomalacia, and immature muscles cause GERD. Unfortunately, the two often work hand-in-hand, and having both laryngomalacia and GERD can aggravate a baby's breathing problems. Laryngomalacia makes GERD symptoms worse, and GERD intensifies laryngomalacia symptoms. If your baby already has a floppy epiglottis, then irritation from stomach acid will make the floppy epiglottis a little red and swollen, making her breathing a bit noisier. Babies with both GERD and laryngomalacia (laryngomalacia combined with GERD is usually diagnosed with a tiny camera by an ear, nose, and throat doctor, who will see a red, swollen, floppy epiglottis) will more likely be treated by making some feeding position changes as well as receiving medications.

If your baby's GERD is severe, with substantial acid and liquid reflux into the throat, it may also be causing nasal stuffiness. The acid and milk/formula will come up and irritate the back of his nose, causing swelling and congestion.

If my baby has GERD that is causing a breathing problem (or aggravating a breathing problem), will she grow out of it?

Most babies with GERD (even if there is a breathing problem as well) grow out of it. As the muscles mature, as the sphincters tighten, and as the stomach expands and can handle more volume at a given feed, GERD symptoms subside. This may start to happen when solids are introduced (typically at the age of six months), or it may continue until the first year. A very small percentage of newborns with GERD will require treatment after the first year.

THE BIG PICTURE

All newborns have some degree of gastroesophageal reflux (GER). The combination of immature muscles, immature sphincters, and closeness of all of the structures means that stomach contents can come back up, either during a feed or soon after. As the muscles 'learn' to move in the right direction, as the sphincters tighten, and as your baby grows, most reflux gradually subsides. However, some babies have more difficulties, and the combination of the milk/formula mixed with the stomach acid can be quite irritating. Some babies with GERD will have symptoms of colic, with pain, arching, and frequent spit-ups or even vomiting. Even without true colic, some babies will have GERD that affects their breathing, especially if there is a breathing problem to begin with (such as laryngomalacia — floppy epiglottis, or a stuffy nose). In these cases, the stomach acid will cause the delicate breathing structures to swell.

Reflux doesn't usually start in the first few days, so it may take several visits with your pediatrician until it is discovered. As with most newborn issues, weight gain is usually a good sign, and will allay any concerns for serious GERD, even if your baby has frequent spit-ups. But frequent spit-ups, discomfort, or breathing problems along with a poor weight gain may be a strong indication to investigate the possibility of GERD. Some pediatricians will recommend a trial of medications, while some may prescribe some tests, which will assess both the presence as well as the severity of any GERD.

DON'T WORRY

If you have a spitter, but she is comfortably feeding and growing, your baby very likely has a 'normal' degree of reflux. Over the next several months, the spitting will reduce as your baby grows. The quantity of the spit-up may sometimes seem like a lot, but remember that a lot of it is mixed with the fluids produced by the stomach itself. Your baby may also have some days with a lot of spit-up, both in frequency and amount, and some days with almost no spit-up at all. This is also a normal variation of the mild degree of reflux that almost all babies have.

WORRY

If your baby has voluminous spit-ups, and seems uncomfortable (crying, arching, or even shows resistance) with feeds, she may have GERD. If these symptoms are associated with poor weight gain, coughing, nasal stuffiness or noisy breathing with blue spells, you should let your pediatrician know. This degree of reflux is usually not seen right after birth, but more commonly in the first four to six weeks after birth.

TO-DO LIST: NEWBORN BREATHING ISSUES RELATED TO FEEDING

1. If your baby's breathing sounds noisy or stuffy during or after feeds, let your pediatrician know. She may not see this during a routine check-up. Ask her to watch you feed your baby if you need to demonstrate what you mean.

2. If your baby is diagnosed with GERD-related breathing problems, try smaller and more frequent feeds, more frequent breaks for burping, and remember to keep your baby in the upright position for at least 20–30 minutes after each feed.

3. Your pediatrician may recommend medications to help your baby settle her GERD symptoms. For the vast majority of infants, these are needed only temporarily, and can usually be phased out between the ages of six and 12 months.

Sources for Newborn Feeding and Breathing Problems:
www.entnet.org/healthinformation/pediatricGERD.cfm
www.entnet.org/healthinformation/laryngopharyngealreflux.cfm
www.infantrefluxdisease.com/infant_acid_reflux

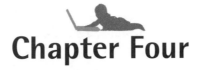

Chapter Four

Back to Sleep and Beyond: SIDS Prevention

Newborns spend a lot of their days (and for your sake, hopefully nights) sleeping — up to 14 to 18 hours per day in the first week, and 12 to 16 hours per day in the first few months. Since they easily spend more than half of their time asleep, it is crucial that this is done safely. The safest (and only) way to have your newborn sleep is **on his back**. In the coming chapter, you will realize how critical this is. In 1992, the American Academy of Pediatrics (AAP) found evidence that newborns who sleep on their stomachs have a significantly higher risk of Sudden Infant Death Syndrome (SIDS). After the AAP made this recommendation public, the rate of SIDS dropped by over 50%. However, SIDS still remains the leading cause of death in young infants, so the emphasis of the importance of 'Back to Sleep' needs to be a continued effort.

My baby loves to be on her tummy, and seems to prefer that position when I put her down to sleep. Is that ok?

No! It is not. 'Tummy time' is great for your baby — it helps build strong neck and shoulder muscles, and helps with her overall physical and cognitive development. This should only be done with direct adult supervision, especially in very young infants. Their upper body strength is very minimal, and they may need help even to keep their head turned to one side, so that they do not face down on a surface. Tummy time should be on a firm, padded surface. A soft mattress or very plush carpet will make it more difficult for your newborn to enjoy tummy time safely. But even if she loves tummy time, you must place her on her **back (not on her**

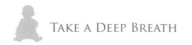

side or stomach) to sleep. By about age four to seven months, babies can roll over on their own. Until that point, they need to be on their backs during sleep.

Why is tummy-sleeping so dangerous? I slept on my tummy as a newborn, and I turned out just fine!

While the majority of us born before 1992 slept on our tummies for most of our infancy, that doesn't necessarily make it safe. I never had a car seat, rarely wore seatbelts, and used mercury thermometers. That doesn't mean I would practice these behaviors with my children, knowing what we know today. New research has proven that the risks of tummy sleeping are significant. One possible risk is that when an infant sleeps on his stomach, there is increased pressure on the jaw, which can compress the upper airway and restrict breathing. Another possibility is that when facing down, the baby is 'rebreathing' his own exhaled air while creating a small, enclosed space around his mouth and the mattress. This 'rebreathing' of carbon dioxide will lead to decreased oxygen and can contribute to SIDS. Some parents have concerns that a baby who sleeps on his back will have a higher likelihood of vomiting and choking. The American Academy of Pediatrics has shown that there is no increased risk of this. However, if your baby has severe **gastroesophageal reflux disease (GERD) or laryngomalacia** (see Chapters Two and Three), your doctor may recommend alternative positioning such as head elevation (but not tummy sleep).

What is the safest way for me to put my newborn to sleep?

There are some very basic practices you can routinely use to put your newborn to sleep. Make sure that these are carried out for anyone else who is helping to take care of your baby. These practices are non-negotiable! They are not lifestyle choices, but life-saving ones. *One in five SIDS deaths occur while someone other than a parent is caring for an infant.* Safe sleep practices need to be fully explained to anyone who will be watching your baby, even if it is just for a brief time for you to get a quick shower or a snooze yourself:

❖ Always place your baby on his back when putting him to sleep, even if he is still awake.

❖ Don't place your baby on his side, as he is more likely to roll on to his stomach than his back.

- ❖ Don't cover his head with a blanket, and don't over-bundle him. A snug wrap or sleep sack is fine.
- ❖ Make sure that your baby's head and neck are comfortably open and in the upright position.
- ❖ If you use a wrap or a swaddle, make sure that your baby's arms are comfortably at his sides, and well secured.
- ❖ If you use a sleep sack (usually these are zip-up sacks with arm holes) make sure that it is the proper size for your baby. If it is too big, it may cinch up and cover your baby's head. If it's too small, his legs will get cramped up and he wont be able to straighten them comfortably.
- ❖ Make sure that the crib has a firm mattress with a well-fitted sheet. Bassinettes and cradles are fine, but make sure they are firm with a well-fitted sheet.
- ❖ Don't place your baby on a chair, sofa, waterbed, or adult bed to sleep.
- ❖ Remove any toys, pillows, cozy blankets, and stuffed animals from the sleeping area before putting your baby to sleep.

My baby sleeps on his back, but now he is eight weeks old and has a flat head!

As the "Back to Sleep" campaign has become the gold standard, we are seeing more and more 'flat heads' (**positional plagiocephaly**). Young infants have very pliable bones in their head, primarily because the **sutures** (openings in the skull bones) have not yet fused, allowing for the brain and skull to undergo tremendous unhindered growth in the first 12 months. Babies who sleep on their backs may develop a flat spot on the back of the head. It is usually easily treatable by increasing tummy time when your baby is awake, or having his head turned to one side or the other during sleep (while remaining on his back). Once your baby is able to roll over (usually between the age of four and seven months), the 'flat head' resolves. If your baby's head shape remains quite flat, or asymmetric, your pediatrician may recommended that you see a type of specialist called a 'craniofacial' specialist. This specialist may recommend that your baby wear a helmet (this looks like a bicycle helmet) to help re-shape the bones of his skull. Helmets are usually worn for all or part of the day, for a period of weeks to months. While this may seem like a nuisance, these helmets are remarkably well-tolerated by young infants, and

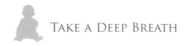

have an extremely high success rate in reversing any head flattening. This is a small price to pay for reducing the rate of SIDS by half.

Is SIDS preventable?

The risk of SIDS has declined significantly ever since the "Back to Sleep" campaign began in the early 1990's. There are factors that increase the risk of SIDS, and factors that lower it, even before your baby is born.

Risk factors for SIDS include:

❖ Smoking, drinking alcohol, or using drugs during pregnancy.

❖ Poor (or no) prenatal care.

❖ Prematurity or low birth weight (this is, of course, for the most part unavoidable, although tobacco use, alcohol consumption, drug use, and poor prenatal care are associated with prematurity and low birth weight).

❖ Tobacco exposure after birth doubles an infant's risk of SIDS.

❖ Overheating from too much sleepwear or bedding.

❖ Stomach sleeping.

Risk Reduction for SIDS:

❖ Back to sleep, firm mattress, no toys, pillows, or loose blankets in the sleep space.

❖ Keep your baby at a comfortable temperature during sleep (a room temperature where you would feel comfortable in light clothing). A baby who is overheated may get into too deep of a sleep, making it more difficult for him to awaken.

❖ Bring your baby to regular well-baby check-ups.

❖ Always check with your pediatrician if you have questions about sleep positioning.

❖ Breastfeeding has been linked to reduce the risk of SIDS. One possible reason is that breast milk helps protect babies from infections. (Some infections such as respiratory illnesses may increase SIDS risk).

❖ Pacifiers during sleep have been linked to lowered SIDS risk.

❖ Having your infant sleep in a crib or bassinette (as opposed to a parent bed) has been linked with a lower risk of SIDS.

My baby sleeps on his back when we are at home, but when we are out, he likes to sleep in a sling or infant carrier. Is this safe sleep positioning?
In 2010, the Consumer Product Safety Commission issued a warning regarding safety of infant carriers after several infant deaths were reported to have occurred in baby carriers. While it is overall safe for your infant to be carried in these carriers, there are several issues you should keep in mind to keep your newborn safe. First of all, these carriers are wonderful ways of enabling your baby and you or anyone caring for your baby to have close contact while you are out and about. The physical closeness that these carriers provide allows your baby to feel similar to how he felt in the womb — even if it is not his mom who is carrying him. Babies feel the warmth of the body, are curled up in a position similar to how they were before they were born, and they also feel the up and down movement of walking while in the carrier. For these reasons, many infants have fantastic naps in these carriers. But here, unfortunately, is where the danger comes in, and where safe positioning for your newborn is crucial when snuggling him up in his sack. First of all, newborns under three or four months of age rely on their tiny noses to breathe (see Chapter One). Make sure that your baby's nose is not pushed up against the cloth of the carrier or up against you directly. Second of all, newborns have very weak neck muscles, and cannot reposition themselves if their neck is bent in a way where their chin is against their chest. Make sure that your baby's neck position is not curled to face downwards. Last but certainly not least, newborns can re-breathe their own carbon dioxide (the substance which we breathe out) if their head is positioned downwards in an enclosed sack. If a baby breathes in his own carbon dioxide, he can become unconscious and stop breathing altogether. When this happens, babies do not struggle or startle, so when you think your baby is sleeping, he may actually not be breathing. Make sure your baby's face is not directly against the material of the sack or your clothes. Keep your baby's head visible to the air, even if the rest of his body is snuggled in the sack.

THE BIG PICTURE

While SIDS remains the number one cause of death in young infants, the "Back to Sleep" campaign, initiated by the AAP, has resulted in a 50% decline in the annual rate of SIDS. I cannot think of a more compelling reason for you to have your newborn sleep on his back. While many babies who succumb to SIDS have no known risk factors and no known reason for this event, extensive research in SIDS has enabled us to educate families about both risk factors as well as risk prevention for SIDS. It is crucial that all caregivers for your baby understand and comply with safe sleep habits for your newborn. 'You slept on your stomach and you're just fine. And besides, it's more comfortable' is not a reason for your baby to sleep on his stomach. This is non-negotiable. And as with all issues, especially in your newborn, when in doubt, ask your pediatrician.

DON'T WORRY

If your newborn develops some flattening of his head from sleep positioning, this can be easily rectified in the early months of life. If it is mild, usually repositioning your baby to either side during wake periods will allow for pliable skull bones to re-shape. Very rarely, babies will need a 'helmet' (this looks like a bicycle helmet), worn for all or part of the day, to help mold the skull bones. These babies, however, usually have head flattening (**plagiocephaly**) soon after birth, not solely from sleeping on their back.

WORRY

If you are putting your baby to sleep on his stomach, you should worry. If you leave loose blankets, plush toys, or pillows in your baby's sleep area, you should worry. If your baby sleeps on a soft mattress, you should worry. If even one caregiver does not know to put your baby to sleep on his back, you should worry. It is not too late to change these practices. Then you will not have to worry!

TO-DO LIST: BACK TO SLEEP AND BEYOND: SIDS PREVENTION

1. It starts before your baby is born — get regular prenatal care, do not smoke, do not drink alcohol, and do not use drugs.

2. Create safe sleep places for your newborn — a crib and/or a bassinette with a tight-fitting sheet. Remove all toys and blankets from the sleep area during sleep.

3. Tummy time is fine, but only in an awake infant under adult supervision. The infant should be on a firm surface such as a floor or a play-mat.

4. Do not expose your newborn to second-hand smoke.

5. Bring your baby to regular well-baby check-ups.

6. Keep your baby's sleep area at a comfortable temperature (one where you would be comfortable in light clothing). Overheating can increase a newborn's risk of SIDS.

7. Swaddling or wrapping (or using a sleep sack) is fine, but make sure that whichever you use fits well — not too snug, but no loose ends.

8. Blankets are not safe to use in sleeping newborns. They can inadvertently cover your baby's head.

9. Always ask your pediatrician if you are not sure about sleep safety.

10. When placing your newborn in an infant carrier, make sure that her face is exposed to air, and is not pressed directly against the material of the sack, her own chest, or your body.

Sources for SIDS:
www.babycenter.com/baby-sleep-safety
www.healthychildcare.org/sids-html
http://kidshealth.org/parent/general/sleep/sids.html
www.sidscenter.org

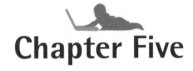

Chapter Five

Wheezing: Can a Newborn Have Asthma?

Wheezing is the turbulent passage of airflow in the **bronchi** (lower windpipe passages) or **alveoli** (tiny air-filled sacs within the lungs). When we think of wheezing, we commonly think of older children with asthma. Newborn wheezing is a bit different. **Asthma** itself is a chronic inflammatory condition of the airways, which usually develops over time. Young infants can have asthma-like symptoms, and this is often termed **reactive airway disease**. The lower airways 'react' to respiratory illnesses or inflammation, thus the term 'reactive' airway disease. In the absence of a respiratory illness, wheezing in a newborn is usually related to lung and/or airway immaturity. In this chapter, I will explain what causes a newborn to wheeze, how to recognize it, and when to call your doctor.

My baby's chest sounds 'congested'. She seems comfortable, but she sounds kind of 'junky', and I can feel some rattling sound when I hold her. What's going on?

Many newborns have some degree of occasional chest congestion. They are learning to coordinate swallowing and breathing, and occasionally some milk/formula or saliva/mucus gets into their windpipe. This wet stuff settles in either their windpipe or lower airways and lungs, and you can hear some rattling. Chest congestion sounds 'wet', and you don't usually hear any high-pitched squeaks from either the throat or the chest. For the most part, a little chest congestion in an otherwise comfortably breathing baby is not a concern. By 'comfortably breathing', I mean no retractions (where the chest, stomach, or neck is caving in with each breath), no rapid breathing

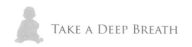

(newborns should breathe 24 to 38 times per minute), and no visible discomfort (arching, crying, skin discoloration). For occasional chest congestion, try holding your baby upright, with her head over your shoulder, as if you were burping her. Tap her back gently. This may encourage some coughing, and help loosen up the wetness. Ideally, she will cough it up into her mouth and then swallow it. If you notice more chest congestion after feeds, make sure your baby stays upright during and after feeding times.

> **NEWBORNS SHOULD BREATHE 24 TO 38 TIMES PER MINUTE.**
> **HOW TO COUNT YOUR BABY'S BREATHS:**
> **HAVE HIM LYING COMFORTABLY, AND COUNT THE NUMBER OF BREATHS FOR THIRTY SECONDS.**
> **MULTIPLY THIS NUMBER BY TWO FOR THE NUMBER OF BREATHS PER MINUTE.**
> **BREATHING RATE CAN GO UP SLIGHTLY DURING A RESPIRATORY ILLNESS OR A FEVER.**
> **IF YOUR BABY IS BREATHING MORE THAN 60 TIMES PER MINUTE, CALL YOUR DOCTOR.**

My five-year-old son has asthma, and my newborn daughter sounds like she's wheezing. Can she have asthma so soon?

Probably not. Or at least not yet. While asthma can run in families, especially if it's the type of asthma related to allergies, very young infants who wheeze do not necessarily have a diagnosis of true asthma. Asthma is a chronic lung condition that leads to swelling in the airways. The airways, in turn, produce more mucus, making it harder for air to pass through the tiny sacs and tubes in the lungs. In a newborn, recognition of a problem and treating that problem is more important than coming to a diagnosis of a chronic condition. 'True' asthma is diagnosed not only by wheezing, but also by lung function tests, whereby the child breathes in and out through a tube into a machine. The machine records the breathing capacity. Needless to say, a cooperative (and older) child is necessary. When you hear wheezing (a whistling sound usually when your baby breathes out, sometimes accompanied by retractions or pulling in of the neck, abdominal or chest muscles), the two most likely causes are lung immaturity or a respiratory illness. This is usually seen more commonly in premature babies, or in full-term babies during an acute respiratory illness. Over 50% of infants have at least one episode of wheezing in the first year, but only one-third of those go on to develop asthma.

Are there certain factors that predispose my baby to have asthma in the future? Is there anything I can do to prevent this?

While one episode of wheezing does not mean that your newborn has (or will have) asthma, there are certain early signs that may keep you on the lookout for asthma in the future. A high risk factor for asthma is tobacco smoke exposure — both before your baby is born and after birth. Before birth, toxins such as nicotine and carbon monoxide are absorbed into the bloodstream of the fetus, leading to higher chance of prematurity (and consequent, lung immaturity), low birth-weight, and inflamed airways. Tobacco smoke exposure after birth is known to be associated with chronic airway inflammation, and higher risk of acute as well as chronic respiratory illnesses. DON'T SMOKE DURING PREGNANCY OR AFTERWARDS. This will lower your baby's risk of asthma. Babies and young children with asthma related to tobacco exposure are also harder to treat — the chronic inflammation in their airways does not respond as well to medications. These children are not only prone to developing asthma, but they are also more prone to developing asthma-related breathing complications requiring hospitalization.

Another risk factor is family history. Newborns whose parents or siblings have asthma or environmental allergies (not allergies to medications or insect stings) have a higher likelihood of developing asthma in the future. Newborns with **eczema** (a skin condition whereby a baby has dry, flaky, itchy skin patches) may also have a predisposition to environmental allergies and asthma in the future.

As far as prevention goes, don't smoke when you are pregnant or after your baby is born, and don't let anyone smoke in your baby's home. If you have a strong family history of asthma, being aware of signs of breathing problems will be the best method of prevention. While you won't necessarily be able to prevent asthma from developing, you can be more proactive when it comes to recognizing early signs of asthma or allergies in your newborn. In the early months of life, a newborn pre-disposed to asthma may be more likely to develop wheezing during a respiratory illness. Recognition by you, and alerting your doctor, will maximize their treatment

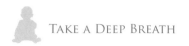

early on, and minimize the likelihood that his symptoms will progress to respiratory difficulties.

My baby was born via Caesarian section. We just brought her home at age four days, and she sounds a little 'wheezy'. Is this normal?

Babies born via C-section (either planned or unplanned), even if full-term, often have a little fluid collection in their lungs. Unlike during a vaginal delivery, babies born via C-section go from a fluid-filled environment directly to an air-filled one relatively 'smoothly', in that they are not squeezed through a tight space. During vaginal delivery, pressure that the muscles of the vaginal walls and pelvic bones put on the baby's ribcage actually helps to clear the amniotic fluid from their lungs and throat before they are delivered. This helps to squeeze out some of the fluid as the baby is being born. In a C-section delivery, the baby is lifted out, without being 'squeezed'. The fluid is suctioned out of their mouth immediately, but their lungs often retain a bit of residual amniotic fluid. Most babies have no visible symptoms from this, as the fluid usually clears in a matter of hours or a day or two. But some may take a little bit longer. Your baby will be checked several times by the hospital's doctors and nurses before he is discharged, so you will probably know about this chest congestion before you go home. A little residual noise is fine, but remember that babies are very good self-regulators, and very good at showing signs of a problem. Even at just a few days old, rapid breathing (more than 60 breaths per minute), blue skin discoloration, or signs of struggling, where the chest, abdomen, or neck muscles cave in, needs immediate medical attention.

My baby was born prematurely. How does this impact his lungs, and what can I expect regarding breathing problems now and in the future?

The degree of lung immaturity really depends on how prematurely your baby was born. For the first seven to eight months of pregnancy, a baby's lungs have not yet developed the capacity to function on their own. A substance called **surfactant** is produced by the lungs between 32 and 34 weeks gestation, which is usually sometime in the eighth or ninth month of pregnancy. Surfactant is a mixture of fats and proteins, and it prevents the tiny airways in the lungs from collapsing onto themselves during inhalation and exhalation. If you know in advance that your baby needs to be born prematurely, doctors can take a small sample of amniotic fluid to determine the amount of surfactant in your baby's lungs, which in turn will determine his lung maturity. If your doctor anticipates that your baby will be born early, she might give you medications to hasten your baby's lung maturity. The most common medication that an obstetrician will administer to hasten lung maturity is **steroids**. This medication promotes the immature lungs to produce surfactant, even before they would normally do so.

After birth, premature babies receive multiple therapies to help with lung development. These therapies may include oxygen supplementation in an incubator, or mechanical **ventilation**, whereby your baby will have a small breathing tube placed into his windpipe. This breathing tube will be attached to a breathing machine, which will help your baby breathe and receive oxygen until he is able to do so on his own.

Some babies who are born prematurely with lung problems may develop **bron-chopulmonary dysplasia (BPD)**. This is more common in very premature babies who are born before 28 weeks, or before you enter your eighth month of pregnancy. It is a chronic lung disorder we see in babies who require long periods of mechanical ventilation (breathing tubes on a breathing machine). The baby's lungs may develop swollen air passages, and he may need to receive oxygen at home, even several months after leaving the hospital. Because of this chronic swelling, these babies are more susceptible to develop lung infections such as bronchitis or pneumonia when they get colds.

> HOME OXYGEN THERAPY FOR BABIES IS GIVEN VIA SMALL PLASTIC TUBING THAT YOU PLACE INTO EACH NOSTRIL. BABY-SIZED TUBES FIT INTO THE VERY FRONT PART OF EACH NOSTRIL.
> THE AMOUNT OF OXYGEN YOUR BABY WILL NEED IS DETERMINED BY YOUR DOCTOR PRIOR TO GOING HOME.
> THE OXYGEN SUPPLY IS IN AN OXYGEN TANK, WHICH IS CONNECTED TO PLASTIC TUBES THAT HAVE THE DIAMETER OF A SMALL DRINKING STRAW.
> YOUR DOCTORS AND NURSES INSTRUCT YOU HOW TO PLACE THE TUBING INTO YOUR BABY'S NOSTRILS, AND HOW TO USE THE DIALS ON THE OXYGEN TANK.

Another respiratory problem that premature babies may develop is called **apnea of prematurity**. Apnea occurs when a baby temporarily stops breathing. This can occur because he temporarily 'forgets' to breathe as a result of an immature nervous system, and is termed **central apnea**. It may also occur as he tries to breathe but the airway collapses. This is termed **obstructive apnea**. Most premature babies, especially those born before 28 weeks, have both central and obstructive apneas, termed as **mixed apnea**. If the episodes of apnea occur several times per day, the baby may remain in the hospital, and will need to be connected to a monitor measuring heart rate, oxygen levels, and breathing rates. These monitors will alarm when there is an apnea event. The hospital staff will be alerted, and will assist the baby's breathing, either by stimulating him (rubbing his back or chest), or giving him some extra oxygen to breathe with an oxygen mask. The oxygen mask is similar to the type you see on airplanes during the emergency demonstrations. Doctors and nurses can also give medications such as **aminophylline** and **caffeine** to stimulate the baby's immature respiratory system and reduce the frequency of central apnea. Most babies 'grow' out of apnea of immaturity by the time they are 'full-term' (equivalent of 40 weeks old, calculated by combining the number of weeks of pregnancy and the number of weeks after birth). For instance, a baby born at 30 weeks will be considered 'full-term' when he is 10 weeks old.

THE BIG PICTURE

Wheezing in newborns is relatively common. At least half of newborn babies will have wheezing at some point. This does not necessarily mean that these babies have asthma, nor does it mean that they will become asthmatic. Wheezing in a newborn baby sounds like a whistling sound when she breathes out. It may be a sign that she is developing a respiratory illness, or it may be transient chest congestion from a Caesarian section birth or from a bit of milk/formula or mucus traveling into the small air passages in the lungs. A brief period of wheezing in a comfortably breathing baby should resolve on its own, but wheezing in a newborn who is struggling to breathe, either by fast breathing or retracting, warrants a call to your doctor right away. Newborns with a family history of asthma may be more predisposed to become asthmatic as well, so these babies should be watched more closely by your pediatrician for early signs of asthma. Babies born prematurely have a higher likelihood of having breathing problems as newborns, due to their lung immaturity. Premature babies with wheezing need close medical attention. They are more susceptible to respiratory illnesses, and more liable for these illnesses to progress to a more serious condition such as pneumonia.

As you will read in every section, and in almost every chapter, you'll read it here again: don't smoke — before or after your baby is born. And don't let anyone smoke near your baby, inside or outside of your home. Not only will it increase your baby's risk of asthma, but it will also make it harder for your baby's asthma to be treated.

DON'T WORRY

If your newborn has very brief periods of wheezing, but is breathing comfortably, eating well, and does not have rapid breathing or struggling, the wheezing noise will most likely resolve on its own. It does not necessarily mean that he has or will have asthma. That said, if your baby's breathing pattern changes, even briefly, and you're not sure what's going on, give your pediatrician a call. It may be something that you can describe over the phone. If there's any concern on your pediatrician's part, she'll ask you to come in for a check.

WORRY

If your baby is wheezing, and at the same time, seems to be breathing rapidly, or is using chest, neck, or abdominal muscles to move air in and out, call your doctor right away, go to the emergency room, or call 911. If your baby shows any signs of blue discoloration of their lips, tongue, or skin while wheezing (**cyanosis**), this is also a reason to get medical attention right away. While various breathing noises are to be expected in a newborn, he should not be struggling to breathe at any time.

TO-DO LIST: WHEEZING: CAN A NEWBORN HAVE ASTHMA?

1. If your baby sounds a little 'junky', with 'wet' breathing, hold him upright, over your shoulder. Remember to support his head. Gently tap on his chest. This will

help loosen any secretions or congestion in his chest, promoting a cough or a burp.

2. Many babies have brief periods of wheezing, with a whistling sound coming from their lungs when they breathe out. As long as this sound goes away on its own, it is not an emergency. Let your doctor know that it occurred, but it may not happen more than once.

3. If you hear wheezing/whistling from your baby's chest, accompanied by rapid breathing rate, cyanosis (blue discoloration), or retractions, seek medical attention right away.

4. If there is a family history of asthma, and you hear wheezing in your newborn, let your pediatrician know.

5. Eliminate any unnecessary risks for wheezing and eventual asthma in your newborn. The number one way to do this is not to expose your baby to cigarette smoke.

6. If there is a family history of asthma or allergies, avoid exposing your baby to potential allergens that are known to trigger asthma attacks in family members, such as dust, pollen, or pets.

Sources for Newborn Wheezing:
www.askdrsears.com
http://kidshealth.org/parent/medical/asthma/wheezing_asthma.html
http://www.healthline.com/health/asthma
www.newbornbabyzone.com/health-safety/10-facts-to-know-about-infant-asthma

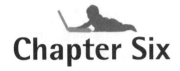

Chapter Six

Respiratory Infections in Newborns

Many newborns will develop a respiratory illness in the first months of life. These are usually viral, are seen more commonly in fall and winter months, in homes with older siblings, or in newborns who were born prematurely. Some respiratory infections in the first three months need not be taken seriously. Nasal congestion, a runny nose, or sneezing are usually nothing to worry about. But coughing, wheezing, yellow/green nasal discharge, or even a low-grade fever (greater than 100.4°F) can indicate a more serious condition. While newborn babies retain some immunity that was transferred from their mother's immune system during pregnancy (this immunity lasts longer if they are breast fed), they have immature airways, and immature immune systems, and are more likely to develop bronchitis or pneumonia from what started out as a cold.

Besides the fact that babies have immature airways, a baby's immunity to viruses and bacteria against which she will be vaccinated has not yet taken place. The first round of immunizations is at the age of two months, and even after your baby receives these vaccines, her immunity to those particular organisms may not be fully developed until weeks or months later, or even after the second or third round of vaccinations at the age of four or six months. A note on vaccinations: while this book will not go into the issues of vaccine controversy, I will simply state that I am pro-immunization. Not only am I pro-immunization, but I also believe that it is important to stay as close to the recommended immunization schedule as possible. Many vaccines require several boosters before a child develops adequate immunity to a potentially life-threatening illness. There is an exhaustive amount of solid research backing the fact

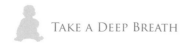

that the benefits of immunizations outweigh the risks. Studies are also now showing that there is a true time limit for the lifespan of a vaccine's ability to confer immunity against certain communicable illnesses. Booster schedules for older children and adults, such as for pertussis, or 'whooping cough', need to be followed as well. These booster vaccines not only protect the child or adult receiving the vaccine, but they also protect young infants who are not yet fully immunized.

VACCINES RECOMMENDED AT AGE TWO MONTHS:
(2010 IN THE UNITED STATES)
(www.cdc.gov/vaccines/recs) (www.aap.org)

❖ Hepatitis B Vaccine (HepB)
❖ Rotavirus Vaccine (RV)
❖ Diphtheria, Tetanus, Pertussis (DTaP)
❖ Pneumococcal (PCV)
❖ Inactivated Poliovirus (IPV)

In this chapter, I will explain the difference between an upper respiratory infection (nose, throat, or sinuses) and a lower respiratory infection (windpipe, bronchi, or lungs) in a newborn baby. Because a newborn's nose is so small, his sinuses are miniscule, and his throat often acts as an open sink to the windpipe, he doesn't always have the ability to prevent viruses or bacteria from entering into his windpipe, bronchi, or lungs. For these reasons, upper respiratory infections in newborns can rapidly lead to lower respiratory infections.

My one-month old has had three days of a runny nose, is coughing once or twice every hour, and is sneezing. How do I know if I should bring him to the doctor?

Young babies can get colds, and they are usually viral and mild. If you have an older child, especially a toddler or preschooler, the likelihood for your newborn developing a cold is even higher. Even if your older child is well, he will act as an amazing 'petri dish', and will bring home 'gifts' of colds and other illnesses from school or playgroups. Make sure that your older child gets into the routine of hand washing (with soap) before touching the baby. It's also not a bad idea to have him change his clothes when he comes home from school. He and/or his friends very likely used his shirt as a tissue, napkin, or towel at some point during the day. However, despite best efforts, or even with no older sibling or no exposure to anyone but you, your newborn may still get a cold.

If your baby does have a cold, much of the treatment can be done at home. Since your newborn is an obligate nasal breather (see Chapter One), he will be pretty uncomfortable if he has a stuffy or runny nose. You should have some nasal saline on hand at home. Spray a few squirts into each nostril ever hour or two. This will help clear the mucus, and it actually flushes out some of the bacteria and viruses that may be infecting your baby's tiny nose. If your baby's nose is very runny, you can use your bulb suction. There are many other types of infant nasal suctions, if your wish to try those as well. Resort to the suction only if his nose is so runny that you can see the mucus dripping out. If your baby is very stuffy but not runny, it's best to hold off on the suction — it will likely just increase the swelling, making him even stuffier. Ask your doctor if it is safe for you to use **oxymetazoline (Afrin®)** nasal spray for your baby. This is a topical decongestant, and it will help shrink his swollen nasal tissues. It can be used as a spray or as a drop (for drops, turn the bottle upside down and drip a few drops into each nostril), and can be used two times per day for up to two days. Remember the rule of twos: Two drops each side, two times per day, for two days. Even though this can be purchased at a drug store or grocery store without a prescription, check with your doctor to see if it is safe for you to use for your baby.

If your baby is just stuffy/runny, with occasional coughing and sneezing, he probably just has a cold that does not need medical attention. Keep him well hydrated with breast milk or formula with normal feeding schedules — it is not recommended to give water to newborns. You can stay ahead of his nasal congestion/runniness by using saline and/or oxymetazoline, and keep him away from anyone who may be ill. However, if he has a fever (100.4°F or above), frequent coughing, wheezing, or breathing difficulties in the setting of what seems like a cold, you should call your doctor, especially in your baby's first six weeks, and even up to three months of age.

My baby has fever and cough. I took her to the doctor and she said it's bronchiolitis. What is this?

Bronchiolitis is a respiratory infection that causes inflammation of the **bronchioles**, which are the small airways that lead from the windpipe to the lungs. It is usually

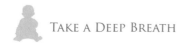

caused by a respiratory virus called **RSV (respiratory syncitial virus)**, and is most commonly seen in the winter and early spring. Bronchiolitis can be caused by other viruses as well, such as **influenza** (flu virus) or **rhinovirus** ('common cold' virus). As a baby's tiny airways swell, they can fill with mucus, making it hard for your baby to breathe. Bronchiolitis is most common in very young babies, because their small airways become more easily blocked than the airways of older infants and children. Most cases of bronchiolitis are mild, and most babies do not require specific medical treatment or hospitalization. However, you should bring your baby to your doctor if she has a cold with coughing, fever, or any breathing trouble. It is often difficult to differentiate a cold, bronchiolitis, and pneumonia in a young infant. That is one of the many reasons that I recommend that you give your doctor a call if your young infant has any fever or cough.

My baby has been coughing for two days, and woke up this morning with a fever of 102°F. I brought him to the doctor and he ordered an X-ray of his chest. My baby was diagnosed with pneumonia and needs to go to the hospital. What should I expect in the next few days?

Because newborn airways are so tiny and fragile, a viral respiratory infection which starts out as a cold can lead to pneumonia in young infants. The small airways (bronchioles) leading to their lungs are not always large enough to clear any mucus that collects during a cold or a cough. This mucus collection may extend into the lungs themselves, resulting in **pneumonia** (a true 'lung' infection). Symptoms of pneumonia usually begin as those similar to a cold — with congestion and mild cough. When these symptoms progress to harsh cough, wheezing, trouble breathing, rapid breathing rate, or retractions, it is possible that the infection has progressed to pneumonia. **Respiratory syncitial virus (RSV)** is the most common cause of bronchiolitis and **pneumonia** (lung infection) in young infants. It results in 90,000 hospitalizations per year and 4500 deaths per year in children under the age of five years in the United States alone. It is a very contagious virus that most of the children worldwide contract at some point before the age of three years. To diagnose RSV pneumonia, your doctor or nurse will place a cotton swab in your baby's nose to obtain some mucus for viral culture sampling. Rapid testing can now be performed within 20 to 75 minutes in a doctor's office to obtain the diagnosis.

Your doctor may also recommend that your baby have an X-ray of her chest. This will help determine whether or not there is an infection in the lungs, and whether one or both lungs are infected. An X-ray of the chest will not necessarily diagnose RSV itself (it can diagnose pneumonia, but not necessarily which virus or bacteria is the culprit), but it will help determine the severity of the infection.

Treatment of the pneumonia depends on the severity of your baby's symptoms. For mild cases, your baby may just be observed in the hospital for a few days. She may receive some humidified oxygen or breathing treatments. She will likely be monitored for her oxygen levels, usually with a lighted sticker on her finger or toe. She will also have monitors measuring her heart rate and breathing rate. She may also receive intravenous fluids if she is dehydrated or is unable to drink.

For babies with severe cases of pneumonia, more intensive monitoring and therapies may be necessary, such as admission to a pediatric intensive care unit to receive breathing treatments, oxygen treatment, a mechanical ventilator (breathing machine), and possibly use of an anti-viral medication (**ribavirin**).

My baby was born two months early. What is the 'pneumonia' vaccine? Why didn't my four-year-old receive it when she was a baby?

While the American Academy of Pediatrics (AAP) does not recommend a 'pneumonia vaccine' to all infants, there is a vaccine to prevent RSV in selected groups of infants. This vaccine, called **palimizuvab (Synagis)**, is given to at-risk infants one time per month during the RSV season (October to May). The vaccine is not recommended for all infants — partly due to the fact that most RSV infections are mild. The other reason is the cost — each vaccine costs about $900. As of 2009, the AAP recommends that the following infants receive Synagis:

1. Children less than two years old with chronic lung disease.
2. Infants born at less than 28 weeks and who are less than 12 months old during RSV season.
3. Infants born between 29 and 32 weeks who are less than six months old during RSV season.
4. Infants born between 32 and 35 weeks who are less than three months old during RSV season and are either attending daycare or have a sibling less than five years old at home.

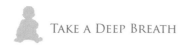
5. Children under two years old with heart or lung disease.

6. Infants born before 35 weeks with neurologic or lung problems.

My baby has a deep, heart-wrenching cough that seems unstoppable.
She is miserable. What could it be?

Severe coughing spells with 'whooping' sounds may be caused by the bacterium, *Bordatella pertussis*, the organism responsible for causing whooping cough, or **'pertussis'**. Pertussis was a disease very commonly seen in the 1930's, with up to 250,000 people contracting the illness per year in the U.S. After routine vaccination against pertussis began in the 1940's, cases of whooping cough declined dramatically. Pertussis immunization is included in the **DTaP** vaccine. The 'P' in the **DTaP** vaccine is for pertussis. DTaP is given at ages two, four, and six months, and then once between 12 and 18 months, followed by a booster at 4-6 years. Children do not develop adequate immunity to pertussis until after the third vaccine, in other words, which is after the age of seven months.

Because immunity from pertussis is not life long, many adolescents and adults will lose their immunity to pertussis, and develop a pertussis infection, or whooping cough. Adolescents and adults who develop a pertussis infection may initially have signs of a mild cold, such as runny nose, low-grade fever, and a mild cough. *It is at this point, before they even know that they have pertussis, that they are highly contagious.* The seemingly benign cold-like illness will progress to a dry, irritative cough with severe coughing spells. Usually these spells are followed by a 'whoop', as the sufferer is gasping in for air. Infants who are not yet fully immunized, which includes all infants under the age of seven months, may be exposed to a teenager or adult with pertussis. Infants who develop pertussis may develop a more severe illness, such as pneumonia and even death from blocked breathing passages. For this reason, it is critical that adolescents and adults, especially those exposed to young infants without pertussis immunity, receive a special pertussis booster called a **TDaP**. This will not only protect the adults and teenagers themselves from developing pertussis, but it will also give critical protection for your baby.

Treatment for pertussis in infants is most successful if begun in the early stages of the disease, with antibiotics and close monitoring of symptoms. However, the 'whooping' coughing spells often don't occur until several days of a minor cold-like illness has developed. Most people are treated successfully with antibiotics, but a young infant may need to be hospitalized, especially if her breathing symptoms are severe, or if her coughing spells are interfering with her ability to drink fluids.

DTaP IS AN ABBREVIATION FOR DIPHTHERIA, TETANUS, PERTUSSIS. TEENAGERS AND ADULTS, ESPECIALLY THOSE EXPOSED TO INFANTS, SHOULD RECEIVE BOOSTERS FOR THIS VACCINE. THE BOOSTER FORM IS CALLED TDaP

THE BIG PICTURE

Upper respiratory illnesses in newborns are oftentimes mild, and most infants develop a cold or cold-like illness sometime in the first months of their life. However, because infants have immature airways and immature immune systems, the window of opportunity to see a doctor is quite small. If your baby has mild stuffiness, clear nasal drainage, sneezing, or a light cough (without fever), you can usually manage this at home, perhaps following a reassuring discussion with your pediatrician. If your baby has any fever over 100.4°F, green or yellow nasal discharge, or a deep cough, call your doctor, or go to an urgent care center or an emergency room. Needless to say (but I'll say it — this is a breathing book, after all), if your newborn baby has ANY signs of ANY breathing trouble, he needs immediate medical attention.

DON'T WORRY

If your newborn is a bit stuffy, with a clear runny nose and sneezing, he likely has the first of many colds to come. You can tell if your baby is ok if she is feeding normally, sleeping normally, and does not have any trouble breathing, aside from the stuffiness. But when in doubt, especially when dealing with a sick newborn, it is always prudent to give your pediatrician a call. You most likely will not need to go to the doctor's office, but describing your baby's symptoms in detail may help your doctor decide whether or not you need to come in for a visit. Another issue to keep in mind is duration of your baby's cold symptoms. The average cold should last three to four days. If the symptoms persist for longer than that, even if they are mild, your doctor may want you to bring your baby in for a check.

WORRY

If your newborn baby has any fever, cough, or trouble breathing, he needs medical attention right away. Seemingly minor illnesses in a young infant can rapidly progress to a more serious illness or infection. This is especially the case in babies born prematurely. Premature babies have airways and immune systems that are much less mature than those of babies born at full-term.

TO DO LIST: RESPIRATORY INFECTIONS IN NEWBORNS

1. For a stuffy nose/clear runny nose, help to keep your baby's nose 'clean' by spraying a few squirts of nasal saline into each side every few hours. While most of the saline solution will come out, it will actually 'flush out' some of the mucus from your baby's nose.

2. Ask your doctor if it is safe to use oxymetazoline (Afrin®) for your stuffy-nosed baby. If so, you can give one or two sprays two times per day for up to two days (Rule of Twos!). If your baby is still stuffy after two days, you must stop this medication. If you don't stop, the medicine will actually make your baby even stuffier.

3. You can use a nasal suction in moderation, but you should limit its use to when your baby has copious mucus draining out of her nose. You will either be given one to take home from the hospital, or you can buy one in the baby section of most pharmacies.

4. If your baby has a fever, call your doctor, even if a fever is his only symptom. If you don't have a thermometer, you should. While rectal temperature is most accurate, you can take your baby's temperature in her armpit. Add one degree to the number from her armpit temperature (in Fahrenheit) to get the 'true' temperature. Ear thermometers are also quite accurate and well tolerated.

5. If your baby has yellow or green mucus draining from his nose, call your doctor. It may just be a sign of a cold, but it also may indicate a bacterial infection. Sometimes green/yellow mucus leads to fever, so it's always a good idea to be one step ahead on this one.

6. If your baby has dry or wet cough, call your doctor. It can sometimes be the earliest sign of a 'lower respiratory' (bronchial/lung) infection.

7. If your baby has any breathing trouble, manifested by coughing, flaring of her nostrils, or retracting (using neck, chest, or stomach muscles for breathing), call your doctor right away. If her breathing trouble comes on suddenly, go to the nearest emergency room or call 911.

Sources for Respiratory Infections in Newborns:
www.dhpe/org/infect/rsv
www.rsvinfo.org
www.pediatrics.about.com/cs/commoninfections/a/rsv_prevention
www.kidshealth.org/parent/infections/lung/bronchiolitis
www.rsvinfo.com/managing/allabout
www.webmd.com/baby/antenatal-corticosteroids-for-fetal-lung-development
www.pediatrics.about.com/cs/commoninfections/a/pertussis
http://www.soundsofpertussis.com/#/whatispertussis

Chapter Seven

Clear the Air for Your Newborn

You've had a beautiful baby shower. The nursery is ready, the clothes are folded, and the latest and greatest light-up, automatic, hermetically sealed diaper pail is plugged in. You took great care of yourself throughout your pregnancy — you took your pre-natal vitamins, ate organically, slept well, cut out caffeine, and would not go to any town unless it was 'smoke-free'. But what now? You've had complete control over your baby's environment throughout pregnancy. Literally. Now that your baby is born, and ready to come home, what can you control? What do you need to control? What is best left out of your control? You live in a house built almost 100 years ago. Should you move? How many layers of lead paint were there before you repainted? Some of your baby gifts were (oh no!) MADE IN CHINA!! Are these gifts coated with lead? Are they safe? You know that you cannot and should not cocoon your baby forever, but you don't want to subject him to harmful chemicals, especially in the first months of his life.

A lot of my friends with newborns have purchased air purifiers for their babies' rooms. Is this necessary? How do they really work?

Air quality in the home, especially one with a newborn baby, is a valid concern. You certainly don't want to increase your baby's risk of breathing problems such as asthma and respiratory infections by having a polluted environment at home. The best ways to minimize risks of 'indoor pollution' is to minimize sources of such pollution. Tobacco smoke is the number one worst, and avoidable, indoor pollutant. Even if the smoker does so outside of the home, the clothes he or she wears carry many of the toxins from cigarette or cigar smoke, potentially exposing a newborn to such harmful chemicals.

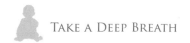

Air purifiers are not absolutely necessary, but some parents do choose to have them at home, especially if there is a lot of dust, old furniture, old carpets, and other family members with asthma or allergies. The most well-known air purifier is a **HEPA (High Efficiency Particulate Air) filter.** A HEPA filter consists of fiberglass fibers that trap very small pollutants and particles in the air. They can trap particles as small as 0.1 micrometer (one hundredth of a millimeter), which accounts for over 99% of air particles, including allergens, mold, pet dander, and dust. Because these filters trap both large and small particles, it's important to change filters on a regular basis. Each brand comes with instructions and recommendations on how often these filters need to be changed.

What else do I need to be concerned about as far as indoor pollutants, besides dust and tobacco smoke?

Volatile organic compounds (VOC's) are chemicals (for example, formaldehyde) that are released by liquids or solids in many homes. They are commonly found in paints, varnishes, and adhesives, and can be released into the air for up to one year from the time they are used. They can affect your baby's nervous system and brain development, so if there is a concern that you may have older furniture or paint, you can purchase a VOC test kit to measure the degree of VOC's in the air. If there are high levels of VOC's in your home, one option is to remove the potential source (that vintage trunk you bought at a garage sale may be better left in your garage). Another is to increase the ventilation in the baby's room. If possible, keep windows and doors open as much as possible before your baby first comes home from the hospital. Air purifiers such as HEPA filters may also help to catch many of the VOC's.

Lead exposure is also a concern. In 1978, Federal law mandated that lead be banned from all paint used in housing. Any home built before 1978 is likely to contain some lead-based paint. Lead-based paint can deteriorate over time, and even more so if the house is undergoing any renovation. As it peels, cracks, or is sanded or scraped, the lead dust particles released can be inhaled, leading to lead toxicity or poisoning. While newborns are not yet at the stage where they will be putting things in their mouth or licking walls, lead-based paint can release lead dust into the air. This is commonly seen from lead-based painted window sills.

In your efforts to ventilate the baby's room, those previously tightly closed windows may be difficult to open. If they have lead-based paint, opening the window can release the paint as a dust, which may be blown into the room. When in doubt, you can have your paint tested for lead. This may be best to do before the baby is born, so that the lead-based paint can be removed, and replaced with lead-free paint. Even wallpaper can contain lead or VOC's, especially if it has been there for many years. It is a good idea to have this tested as well.

THE NATIONAL LEAD INFORMATION CENTER CAN BE CONTACTED AT 1-800-424-LEAD OR HTTP://WWW.EPA. GOV/LEAD

Testing for lead and VOC's can be done by a certified Inspector or Risk Assessor, or you can purchase a home test kit to detect lead in paint, soil, and dust. However, the home test kits are not considered to be as reliable as a certified assessment. The National Lead Information Center provides federal regulations and guidelines on home lead testing and management.

Is it ok to have carpet in my baby's bedroom?

Carpeting is fine, but make sure that it is kept clean. If it's a newly purchased area rug, it's best to air it and the padding out before you lay it down. There are very few non-toxic rugs produced, and most contain VOC's. Airing it out and leaving the windows of the room open for a few days will help in removing many of the toxins. Babies are also especially sensitive to dust particles, and the fibrous nature of carpets and rugs causes them to act like sponges for indoor and outdoor air pollutants. Synthetic cleaning products may add more toxins to the carpet, so it's best to use a non-toxic cleaning product. When choosing a cleaning product, beware of seemingly safe 'buzz' words such as 'eco-friendly' or 'natural'. These may or may not have any bearing on what the product actually contains. It is more important to steer clear of products with labels stating 'Danger', 'Poison' or 'Flammable', which tend to have the highest levels of toxins. Products with labels such as 'Caution' or 'Warning' are usually less toxic. Plant-based materials are much safer than petroleum-based ones, and products containing chlorine bleach and ammonia tend to cause the most damage if inhaled, touched, or swallowed.

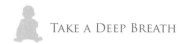

Some vacuum cleaners contain HEPA filters as part of their filtration systems. This gives the best chance of removing small particles from the carpet or rug, without having to add any chemicals to the cleaning process.

We found a beautiful crib at an antique store. If we get it re-painted, is it safe for our newborn?

Beautiful though it may be, it is probably not safe for your newborn, unless the nineteenth century designer was thinking ahead about Consumer Product Safety Commission guidelines. There are now regulations for both cribs and frames, which definitely did not exist in the days of yore. As far as the frames go, the slats need to be no more than 2½ inches apart, to minimize the risk of a newborn's head getting trapped between them. No lead paint can be used on the crib. And as of 2011, there is new concern about drop-down sides for cribs at all, due to risk of accidental drops of the sides resulting in limb injuries or strangulation.

I also recommend that you purchase a new crib mattress. The inner material can be foam or spring, but it should be firm, and it should fit snuggly into your crib frame. Make sure that you purchase one or two water-proof mattress liners. Even though you will feel that you are changing your baby's diapers round the clock, there will be plenty of times when your baby will wet through her diaper and clothes, or will vomit, etc. A waterproof mattress liner is more important than an 'anti-microbial' crib mattress that some manufacturers push. Keeping your baby's crib mattress clean by keeping it lined has more value than an unnecessary item.

Crib bumpers, those lovely, plush pillow-type liners that are often sold with luxury crib bedding sets, are also considered to be dangerous to newborns. There have been reports of newborns' heads getting stuck under these pillows, leading to suffocation. Most pediatricians advise against these.

After having said the above, I must say that the issue of crib safety has one of the most rapidly changing guidelines and recommendations. When my daughter was born, crib bumpers were a must, to prevent her arms and legs from getting stuck in the wooden crib slats. Four years later when my son was born, crib bumpers were nearly outlawed, as the risks of his head getting stuck under one of them frightened me enough to ditch them, much as I loved the little boat and fishy theme I had bought to match his sheets. I breathed a huge sigh of relief when I realized that somehow my daughter survived her life-threatening crib bumpers. And I now breathe a huge sigh of relief knowing that somehow my son survived his now life-threatening drop-down side crib rails. I have no doubt that crib safety will continue to evolve. Perhaps my grandchildren will have to sleep on a hardwood floor, with no crib at all.

THE BIG PICTURE

In general, air quality is often put by the wayside in planning for your new baby. While it is hard to have much control over outdoor air quality (aside from living in a rural area, and being environmentally conscientious yourself), you do have some control over your baby's indoor air quality. The obvious control you have is to keep your baby away from any tobacco smoke or tobacco smokers. There are innumerable studies showing that children who were exposed to tobacco smoke as infants are at a higher risk for developing asthma and chronic lung diseases than those who were not.

Air toxins besides cigarette smoke can also be detrimental to your baby's breathing, such as volatile organic compounds (VOC's) and lead emitted from certain paints, furniture finishes, and carpets. The easiest and least expensive way to clear your baby's room of indoor air toxins is to provide adequate ventilation. This will help remove some of the VOC's, but not lead. Lead-based paint or wallpaper needs to be removed.

When purchasing your baby's crib, or receiving it as a gift or a hand-me-down, check with your pediatrician regarding current safety guidelines for both the frame and the mattress. If you have more children in the future, it is likely that these guidelines will change by the time they are born.

DON'T WORRY

If you live in a home where you know that the paint is lead-free, and there are no smokers, you are in great shape for giving your baby the cleanest air possible. Presence of other chemical compounds found in carpets and furniture can be analyzed, especially if the furniture is antique or vintage. A brand new area rug is best if aired out for a few days before placing in the baby's room. Don't worry if you do not have an air purifier. While they are excellent products that filter out the majority of air particles, there is no data to support that babies who DO NOT have air purifiers are at risk for breathing problems. Certainly, if there is a strong family history of asthma and environmental allergies, a good air purifier can minimize your baby's chance of being exposed to such irritants that predispose him to these disorders.

WORRY

If anyone smokes around your baby, or smokes before being around your baby, they are putting him at risk for developing respiratory problems down the line, including asthma, chronic lung infections, sinus infections, throat infections, and even ear infections (ear infections are considered respiratory infections, as the inside of the ear is connected to the back of the nose).

If there is lead-based paint in the house, or if the window sills contain lead-based paint, the lead dust can become airborne, and can cause not only breathing problems, but also lead poisoning, which can cause damage to your baby's developing nervous system. If you are concerned about lead levels in your home, have this assessed before your baby is born.

TO-DO LIST: CLEAR THE AIR FOR YOUR NEWBORN

1. Don't smoke.

2. Don't expose your baby to people who smoke.

3. If you are concerned that the paint, wallpaper, or window sills have lead, get them checked well in advance of your baby's birth. That will give you time to strip the paint/wallpaper, air out the room, and get it repainted (or wallpapered).

4. If you have a new area rug or carpet, air it and the pad out for a few days before laying it down in the baby's room.

5. Air out the room as much as possible before the baby comes home. Make sure that the window sills are not filled with dust/paint particles. These may contain lead from old paint jobs.

6. Air purifiers are great products to aid in filtering air particles. If other family members have environmental allergies or asthma, it is reasonable to purchase an air purifier for the baby's room. These, however, are not necessary. It is more important to minimize/remove obvious toxins such as lead-based paint and tobacco smoke than to purchase an air purifier.

7. Crib safety is an ever-changing issue. Check with your pediatrician regarding current safety guidelines regarding materials and crib construction. It is best to do this BEFORE you buy one. They can get pricey, as can the accessories.

Sources for Clearing the Air for Your Newborn:

http://www.epa.gov/lead

1-800-424-LEAD

www.organicconsumers.org

www.entnet.org/healthinformation/second-hand-smoke-and-children

http://baby-organic-products.com

www.ecoevaluator.com/lifestyle/health-and-safety/green-your-home-before-the-baby

www.air-purifiers-america.com

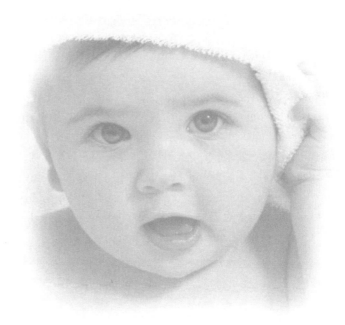

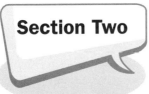
Section Two

THREE MONTHS TO ONE YEAR

This age group is less fragile than the newborn group. Babies at this stage are more robust, interactive, alert, playful, and mobile.

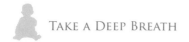

While many concerns of newborn breathing may persist, babies in this age group are better equipped to manage some minor blockages or variations in breathing patterns. However, new breathing problems and variations arise in this age group. Again, working from nose to lungs, in this section, I will give tips on preventing and treating nasal stuffiness and colds, I'll explain why funny 'back of the throat' noises of the newborn period may actually become 'noisier' at this stage, and I'll give you tips on how to recognize an emergency if your baby is having trouble breathing. I will provide life-saving tips to prevent your child from choking on unsafe foods, and I'll give you suggestions on promoting 'safe' feeding during these exciting months of your baby's first year. I will also explain why babies get so many colds (and why that is ok!). I'll also describe some of the more concerning respiratory infections specific to this age group. Some babies begin to develop chronic problems, more than just the occasional cold, and in this section, I will explain why your doctor may recommend 'breathing treatments' (nebulizers) in some situations. If faced with this, I will give you tips on methods of using these treatments, even on the squirmiest eight-month old three times per day!

Chapter Eight
Stuffy Nose in Babies: What's Up There?

After about the age of three or four months, babies 'learn' how to breathe through their mouth. The complex reflex to open their mouth when their nose is stuffy develops during these months, and the riskiness of a stuffy-nosed infant becomes a concern of the past. However, nasal stuffiness in older infants can still be frustrating, if not dangerous. It's often hard to tell if your baby is stuffy from being sick, or because she is just plain stuffy. Oftentimes babies will have congestion without a runny nose — the two do not necessarily go hand in hand. Stuffiness in this age group can be caused by dry air, irritants such as dust, or infections.

My eight-month-old seems stuffy all the time, but he doesn't seem sick. What could this be caused by?
There are many potential sources of nasal stuffiness in infants. The best way to break these down are 'internal' causes and 'external' causes. 'Internal' causes are those that are part of your baby's body. These are actually somewhat uncommon in this age group. There are rare structural variations, such as small nasal passages, **deviated nasal septum** (extremely rare in infants, unless there was nasal injury), or **adenoid** enlargement. The **adenoids** will be a major area of discussion in Section Three (ages one to five years). Adenoids are lymph node tissue (similar to the **tonsils**) that are located at the very back of the nose (you cannot see them directly). They tend to undergo a period of growth between ages one and five years, and may contribute to nasal congestion, sinusitis, and snoring. Very rarely, babies under 12 months will have enlarged adenoids, causing nasal stuffiness, but this is not at all common.

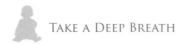

More commonly, babies in this age group will have an 'external' source of nasal congestion. These sources may include dry air, irritants, allergens, or even foreign objects. Excessively dry air, especially in the winter months, when you have your heater on, can reduce production of nasal secretions, leading to crusting and stuffiness. Ambient irritants, such as cleaning solutions, dust, cigarette smoke, or outdoor pollutants, may cause the nasal tissues to swell, leading to congestion. Allergens certainly can cause nasal congestion. However, true 'environmental allergies' are usually not the cause at this age. Babies' immune systems are still immature. Allergies are caused by a 'hyperimmunity' to a certain substance. Such 'hyperimmunity' usually does not develop until later in childhood (ages four or five).

Foreign objects in the nose are also more commonly a concern in older children (toddlers are notorious for this). But if your baby has obvious congestion on ONE SIDE of her nose, with green or yellow drainage on that one side, it may be a sign that she has placed something up there. If you didn't see it happen, or can't see the object yourself, do not be tempted to dig it out. Have your pediatrician take a look. If he can't remove it, he may refer you to an ear, nose, and throat specialist.

My six-month-old has a bad cold. My pediatrician said it was viral, and that she didn't need any antibiotics. But she is miserable. What can I do?

Colds in this age group can be quite distressing, even if your baby is beyond the 'danger' months of illnesses. Most babies will have at least six colds in his first year, so expect at least a few. Colds (usually caused by a multitude of over 100 types of 'cold' viruses) are much more common than bacterial infections or the flu. Symptoms of a cold in a baby will seem worse than those of an older child or an adult, mainly because they are dealing with a much smaller nose, and a much weaker immune system. Babies with colds also often have some feeding difficulty, as it is hard for them to coordinate feeding and swallowing when their nose is so blocked.

When your baby has a cold, with a stuffy/runny nose, there are some home remedies you can try. Saline nasal spray (this is over-the-counter, and all strengths and bottle sizes are safe at all ages) should be used regularly. By 'regularly', I mean as often as you and your baby can tolerate. Put the nozzle of the bottle inside your baby's nostril, then give the bottle a good squeeze. Do this when your baby is upright. Most of the saline will drip out, but some will get up there and flush things out. Most babies HATE this (and so, therefore, will you). But this one is really worth trying, several times. It's even good to use on a regular basis. By 'regular' in this sense, I mean every day. Use of saline nasal spray on a daily basis has shown to cut down the severity, duration, and frequency of colds in both kids and adults. There's no chemical in it, it is not addictive, and really does work. Another option for a baby with a cold is **oxymetazoline** spray (commonly known as **Afrin**®). This is a topical decongestant that can also be bought over-the-counter. For this one, you should definitely check with your pediatrician. Although it is safe in most newborns, it is a drug, so make sure that your pediatrician is fine with it. It works by shrinking the swollen nasal tissues and reducing the amount of mucus produced. If you do use it, you can use it as a spray (similar to nasal saline) or as a drop. Its use, unlike saline, really needs to be limited. No more than *two* sprays, *two* times per day, for *two* days. (2-2-2). The reason for this is that oxymetazoline can quickly cause a 'rebound' effect, whereby the nasal tissues can become even more swollen and congested if you use the spray beyond the recommended few days. Sometimes adults can actually become addicted to oxymetazoline. As is the case with many drugs used in excess, if you use the spray too much, you will need more spray in order to have any benefit. Your nose will just become stuffier, and you will need yet again more spray, and so on. Occasionally, doctors will even need to place patients who are addicted to such decongestant sprays on oral steroid medications to break the cycle. Not fun, so don't try this on yourself, or on your baby!

Babies with colds may also be miserable because it's hard to sleep with a stuffy/ runny nose. Try to keep her head elevated as much as possible during these periods. At this age, it may be tricky to prop up the head of the crib with a wedge or pillow — most babies are pretty mobile at night, and she may end up with her feet elevated and her head downhill. If she is congested to the point of being unable to sleep, try having her sleep in an infant swing, at least for naptime. You can also use the infant car seat for sleep at home. Just remember to place the car seat on the floor. Babies at this age are strong enough to flip their car seat, with them in it. Don't put her in it on the kitchen table, your bed, or a chair. Flipping a car seat off a table with a baby in it — strapped in or not — is not a good thing.

Yet another reason your baby may be miserable is that she may have a hard time feeding. If your baby is eating solids, she may lose some interest during a cold. Don't be too concerned about this, and expect some temporary regression in the food

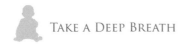

department. The most important thing is to keep her well-hydrated, even if she doesn't have a fever. Keep to her regular feeding schedule as much as possible, but don't be too frustrated if she will have no part of that. If she will not take breast milk or formula, you can try infant hydration drinks such as Pedialyte®, or you can try diluted apple juice or white grape juice. The sweetness might be quite soothing to her, and she will feel better after drinking. Be patient — your baby who normally chugs her bottle in three minutes may take a long time to drink when she's sick.

Humidifiers also help with colds, especially if your baby has a cold in the winter, when the dry heat is on. Make sure you clean your humidifier according to your particular package instructions and recommendations, and make sure you put in enough water to keep it going all night. If your baby is crawling or walking, or if you have older children, keep it out of their reach. Some of the humidifiers get quite hot, and the steam can cause a bad burn. Chest rubs (such as Vicks[R]) are not recommended for babies, and show no evidence of reducing nasal inflammation or drainage in infants. They can even cause skin damage to your baby. Nasal suctioning with bulb suctions or nasal aspirators is often helpful, but I would recommend this only if there is copious mucus coming out. If there is a little nasal discharge, but mostly congestion, suctioning will only lead to more swelling and discomfort. Sometimes using a few squirts of saline nasal spray followed by gentle suctioning of any mucus or saline that you can see dripping out is a good option. You can use saline nasal spray as many times per day as your baby (and you!) can tolerate.

My seven-month-old has had several colds, but this one seems much worse. How do I know if it's more than a cold?

You've become seasoned at managing your baby's colds. But now something is different. Whether it's because he has a fever, has a horrible cough, or is just not 'himself', if it's anything that seems 'different', call your doctor right away. What do you mean by 'different'? you may ask. 'Different' can include any of the following:

- ❖ Fever greater than 102°F for more than one day
- ❖ Fever greater than 101°F for more than three days
- ❖ Fewer wet diapers for one day, or no wet diaper for half a day
- ❖ Ear pain
- ❖ Red eyes or eye discharge

* Cough for one week
* Green or yellow nasal discharge for two weeks
* Just doesn't seem 'right'

Many of these symptoms can be signs of a 'secondary' infection, meaning what was a 'primary' viral cold is now a 'secondary' bacterial infection — either an ear infection, a sinus infection, an eye infection, a throat infection, or a lung infection. Your child may or may not need antibiotics, but he definitely needs to be seen by his doctor. Until you see the doctor, keep doing what you were doing for his cold — humidification, saline nasal spray, plenty of fluids to drink, and gentle suctioning if needed. *Do not give your baby over-the-counter cough and cold medications.* The Food and Drug Administration (FDA), as well as the Consumer Product Safety Commission (CPSC) have deemed that these medications, which contain ingredients such as phenylephrine or pseudoephedrine, can cause serious side effects in infants and children.

If your baby has a fever, you can give **acetominophen** (Tylenol®) every four to six hours. If your baby is over six months old, you can also give **ibuprofen** (Motrin®/Advil®) every six hours. For high fevers, you can alternate one of these (acetominophen OR ibuprofen) every three hours. In this scenario, your baby would receive a fever medication every three hours, but each one would only be given every six hours. Check with your pediatrician before beginning such a regimen. If you have an appointment to bring your baby in, keep a written record of the medications you have given (with the times given), as well as what your baby's temperature has been, when he drank and how much, and how often he has had wet diapers. This is good to do with illnesses in general, even if you don't have an appointment to see your doctor that day. As frazzled as you think you are with all that comes with a baby and a busy schedule, managing a schedule of a sick baby will make your seemingly organized head spin. Here's an example of a chart, to help both you and your doctor keep things straight:

7am	Temp 103°F	Tylenol®
8am	3 oz juice	Dry Diaper
10am	Temp 102°F	Motrin®
11am	2 oz formula	Diaper slightly wet
1pm	Temp 103°F	Tylenol®
2pm	Doctor's appointment	

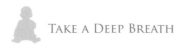

> **FOR HIGH FEVERS IN BABIES OVER THE AGE OF SIX MONTHS, ACETOMINOPHEN (TYLENOL®) *OR* IBUPROFEN (MOTRIN® OR ADVIL®) CAN BE GIVEN EVERY THREE HOURS TO KEEP THE FEVER DOWN.**

I think my 11-month-old stuck something up her nose.
What should I do?

In most cases, do not panic. There is really only one object in the nose that needs absolute emergency medical attention, and that is a *battery of any kind* (most commonly, these are disc batteries we use in watches, cameras, and toys). Batteries can leak chemicals, as well as produce an electric current, that causes rapid damage to any tissues in its contact — be it the mouth, the nose, the throat, or even the ear. These substances can cause permanent damage in a matter of hours. HOWEVER, the most common objects that babies and children stick up their noses are tissues, followed by food, plants, seeds, and toys. It is a rare occurrence in this age group — babies do not have the dexterity to stick small objects in such a small place, and they are more interested in putting things in their mouths than in their noses. But if you do think you saw your baby put something in her nose (and you can't see the object), it's best to have your doctor check it out. Digging around in there yourself will only irritate the area, possibly push the object in further, and make your baby much less likely to cooperate for a doctor's exam. In some instances, you wont witness your baby putting something in her nose, but you may notice that one nostril is stuffy, draining yellow or green mucus, or is giving off a foul smell. All of these signs may indicate an object in the nose. Again, tissues are the most common, and are the most likely to be lodged up there for weeks on end. I've even seen babies who've been diagnosed with 'sinusitis', and placed on antibiotics, when all they needed was a stinky tissue removed. If your baby has nasal symptoms only on one side, consider having her checked for an object in her nose.

My baby seems stuffy in the mornings, and sneezes a lot.
Can he have allergies? Could it be a dairy allergy?

Certainly, babies can have environmental and food allergies, but they are a bit trickier to detect in young infants. Their immune system is not yet developed, so they may not 'test' positive for the allergens at issue. However, if there is a known family history of environmental allergies, it is more likely that your baby may be prone to allergies as well. The 'scratch tests' for specific allergens are not accurately performed until the age of four to five years. There are, however, blood tests that can be performed at younger ages, both for environmental as well as for food allergies. Some of these tests simply measure certain levels of allergy-related substances in the blood. **IgE**, or Immunoglobulin E, is the antibody associated with the type of allergic response one develops to such allergens as pollen, dust, or some foods such as peanuts. **Eosinophils** are a type of white blood cell. These are always present, but usually in very small amounts. Elevation of either IgE or eosinophils may indicate that your child has the potential to develop environmental allergies.

Other blood tests are able to detect specific allergies that a baby may have to certain substances. These tests are called '**RAST**' tests. RAST is an abbreviation for **RadioAllergoSorbent Test**. It is a blood test that is used to determine to what substance a person is allergic. It is different from a skin scratch test, which determines how allergic your child is to a particular substance, indicated by the reaction his skin has to a specific allergen when placed ('scratched') in tiny amounts under his skin. Some advantages of the RAST test over the skin test are that it can measure a full range of allergens, and can detect the level of IgE in the blood directed against suspected allergens. RAST testing can be performed in babies as young as six months old. Skin testing, usually reserved for older children (over four or five years), is in some ways more specific, as it will show the degree of actual allergic response to suspected allergens. In skin testing, a tiny amount of allergic material, such as dust or pollen, is prepared as a liquid. A tiny scratch in the skin is made, with a sharp instrument containing the substance in question. If the area becomes swollen, it indicates that the person is allergic. The degree of skin swelling is related to the degree of allergy to that particular substance. A RAST test showing high IgE to an allergen may not mean that there is actually an allergic response if your child is exposed to that substance. For instance, if your child has a positive RAST test to pollen, it may not mean that he will actually display an allergic reaction when exposed to pollen. Skin testing is more accurate in determining the degree of allergic reaction.

Food allergies (specifically milk/dairy allergy) can also be present in the baby's first year. Even if your baby is being breast fed, he may be allergic to milk proteins (although breast fed babies are much less likely to develop milk allergies than formula-fed babies). A milk allergy occurs when your baby's immune system 'sees' the milk proteins as 'foreign' irritants, thereby 'fighting' them off with an allergic reaction. Most milk allergy symptoms occur before the first birthday, and are slow in onset. Symptoms may include loose and/or bloody stools, vomiting, irritability, or skin rashes, but not nasal stuffiness. Rapid-onset symptoms are rare, but may include wheezing, hives, bumps on the skin, or bloody diarrhea. Milk allergies very rarely cause the severe reaction one sees with other foods such as peanuts. Diagnosing a milk allergy will involve your doctor taking samples of blood and stool from your baby, or by seeing how your baby fares after stopping milk for a short period of time. If your baby does have a milk allergy and is breast feeding, you will need to limit your dairy intake, as milk proteins that you ingest can enter your breast milk. If your baby is formula-fed, you may be asked to switch to a soy-based formula for your baby. If your baby cannot tolerate soy proteins either, there are several hypoallergenic formulas that are better tolerated. DO NOT give your baby goat's milk, sheep's milk, rice milk, or almond milk before his first birthday. Goat's milk and sheep's milk may not be sufficiently pasteurized, predisposing infants to serious infections. Rice milk may not have sufficient nutrients, and almond milk may have allergens similar to those in other nut products.

THE BIG PICTURE

In the first year of life, there are many possible reasons for a stuffy nose. Most commonly, the cause is a cold. Parents are usually not prepared for the frequency of colds in the early years. Babies can get up to ten colds per year, especially if there is an older sibling at home, or if they attend a daycare. The average cold lasts three to four days, so your baby may have a stuffy nose from a cold for up to 20–25% of the year! Less commonly, babies can have early signs of environmental allergies, such as allergies to dust, pets, or pollen. Food allergies such as milk allergies do not usually appear as nasal stuffiness. Many parents feel that reducing or cutting dairy from their child's diet will reduce nasal stuffiness. While dairy products can certainly increase mucus production, they are not necessarily the source of congestion, and there is no reason to completely cut them from your child's diet. The benefits of the vitamins, minerals, and proteins in dairy products far outweigh the nuisance of nasal congestion. The one instance where you should consider reducing dairy (or formula) intake is while your baby is in his crib or bed. If your baby takes a bottle of milk or formula in his bed or crib, his flat positioning while drinking (followed by falling asleep, when it is even harder to clear his throat) can cause more nasal stuffiness, more mucus production, and more congestion. It's also bad for his dental health, even before his teeth have come through. Milk has a surprisingly high sugar content, and this sugar becomes sticky when left in the mouth of an almost-sleeping baby. Feed your baby upright, keep him upright (even if he falls asleep upright), and then put him down.

DON'T WORRY

If your baby has a cold, with a stuffy and/or runny nose, but seems to be eating and/ or drinking relatively well, has wet diapers, and does not have a fever, there is no reason to worry. It is likely one of the many colds that your baby has had or will have. While your baby may be a bit miserable (which, by definition will mean that you will be just as miserable), it is not a serious situation. Keep as much nasal saline spray going as you can, keep your baby hydrated, and use a humidifier in the baby's room during naps and at night. If your baby is chronically stuffy, it may not be a cold, but is usually no reason to worry. You may want to have your pediatrician check for allergies. Many babies at this age will not have allergies, but they will have a stuffy nose nonetheless. They still have tiny nasal passages, so any irritant or mild congestion may make them uncomfortable.

Most babies after about the age of six to eight months are quite 'oral', and, once they start grasping with their own hand, they will put things in their mouths. However, occasionally young infants will put things in their nose. If you think there is an object such as a tissue, a bead, or a piece of food in your baby's nose and you CANNOT see it, let the doctor take a look.

WORRY

If your baby is stuffy/runny, and also has a fever, is not drinking, is not having wet diapers, and seems irritable and/or lethargic, call your doctor right away. *If you think your baby has put a battery of any kind in her nose, seek medical attention right away.*

TO-DO LIST: STUFFY-NOSE IN BABIES: WHAT'S UP THERE?

1. If your baby seems stuffy most of the time, without necessarily being sick, try using nasal saline regularly (a few squirts in each nostril, with your baby upright, before feeding and naptime).

2. If your baby has a cold, saline is still a great option. Cold medication (even over–the–counter cold medication) is not safe for infants, unless it is specifically prescribed by your doctor.

3. If your baby's cold gets worse, where she has fevers, is not drinking or having wet diapers, or if she seems irritable or lethargic, call your doctor. It may be a bacterial infection such as an ear infection, bronchitis, or pneumonia.

4. If allergies run in your family (not medication allergies, but allergies such as those to dust, pollen, or pets), and your baby seems stuffy most of the time, or sneezes frequently, consider having him evaluated for allergies.

5. Noses are not pockets. It will take your child at least three to five years to realize this. If your baby sticks something in her nose, it needs to come out. If it's a battery, it's an emergency. For all other nasal objects, call your doctor, but don't panic.

Sources for Stuffy-Nosed Babies:
www.entnet.org/healthinformation/stuffynose
www.kidshealth.org
www.mayoclinic.com/health/common-cold-in-babies

Chapter Nine
Throaty Noises and Stridor

Chances are, if your baby had some noisy breathing in the first three months, this may continue until his first birthday. By now, you've probably had your doctor (or a specialist) figure out what the noise is from. However, you now have an active baby, whether he's starting to roll onto his stomach, crawl, walk, or just giggle. With more activity comes more rapid, deep breathing, which in turn may bring more noise. **Stridor** is the harsh 'musical', squeaky sound that you hear when your baby is making that noise. It can be heard either when your baby breathes in (**inspiratory stridor**), when your baby breathes out (**expiratory stridor**), or when your baby breathes in and out (**biphasic stridor**). Being able to describe which type your baby has is very helpful for your doctor's evaluation, in that it helps to determine from what part of the air passage the noise is coming. Chronic stridor in a baby who is growing, not struggling to breathe, and is sleeping and eating comfortably, is usually not a concern, and most likely it will start fading by the first birthday. SUDDEN stridor, or sudden worsening of stridor, needs to be attended to right away.

One possible explanation for sudden stridor is a choking episode — on either a toy or food. Babies at this age are very 'oral', and will put all that they can in their mouths. Babies ages 10 to 36 months are most likely to choke on food objects or toys, so it's a great idea to start thinking about what your baby has access to, especially in your kitchen, play areas, and bathrooms.

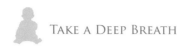

My nine-month-old was diagnosed with moderate laryngomalacia (floppy epiglottis) when he was two months old. Why, if he's older, does the noise he makes sound worse?

Laryngomalacia (see Section One, Chapter Two), is a condition whereby the baby is born with 'soft' cartilage (instead of 'stiff' cartilage) at the top of the airway. The **epiglottis**, which is the leaf-like structure that opens when your baby breathes and closed when your baby eats, can be a little too soft. In this instance, the epiglottis flops closed when your baby breathes in (**inspiratory stridor**), making it sound like a squeaking, or clicking sound. Most babies grow out of this (the epiglottis firms up) at or before the age of 12 months. However, a few things happen before that. One is that the epiglottis sometimes grows more rapidly than it stiffens up. In this case, the noise will get worse before it gets better. In general, the noise peaks at about age six to nine months, after which it gradually gets better. A second issue is that a nine-month-old baby is much more active than a newborn. He is sitting, interacting, and may even be crawling and rolling around on the floor during playtime. This increased activity requires him to breathe more quickly, and to breathe more heavily. These are the times when you may notice more noise. Think about how you are breathing when you are reading this, as opposed to how you are breathing when you are playing with your baby, pushing the stroller, walking a flight of stairs, or even laughing. Your rate and depth of breathing can go up by 25%. So can your baby's when he is more active. If your baby's noise is louder, but he is growing, is playful, is feeding well, and does not seem to be struggling, there is no need to be concerned. It is part of the normal progression of laryngomalacia, and it usually means that it is beginning to go away. If you notice a sudden change in his noisy breathing, or if he is beginning to seem uncomfortable, is having trouble eating, or seems unable to play as a result of the breathing issue, have your doctor check it out — right away if there is a sudden change.

My five-month-old has mild laryngomalacia, but now she has a cold and is really struggling.

Mild laryngomalacia alone is not a concern, and a mild cold by itself is not a concern, but when the two come together, it can be a challenge. If your baby already has a little bit of floppiness in her throat, and then develops a stuffy nose, she may really start to struggle. Most likely there will also be some post-nasal drainage of mucus into the throat, making her throat blockage worse. If your baby has even mild laryngomalacia and develops a cold, you will need to have a higher level of concern than otherwise. This means giving your doctor a call, even if your baby has what would normally be a mild cold. You will also need to put more effort to keep her his nose clean (either by nasal saline, and/or by suctioning). She may need to sleep upright, either in a car seat or infant swing, until the cold passes.

My 11-month old bit into a piece of raw carrot. She coughed and seemed to be choking, but seemed fine right afterwards. Do I need to do anything?

YES! You have entered the 'everything I see goes in my mouth, and I'm quick' stage. Raw vegetables are a no-no for infants under one year. Babies at this age have neither the coordination, patience, nor molars to properly chew and swallow hard foods such as raw vegetables, skinned fruit, nuts, or seeds. When a baby has a choking episode and then seems 'fine', there are a few possibilities of what's happened: (1) she choked on it, coughed it out, and then swallowed it; (2) she choked on it, it went down her windpipe, and the object is now resting in an area beyond the windpipe (towards one lung), enabling her to seem comfortably breathing; (3) she choked on it, and then spit it out. Possibilities 1 and 3 are the most ideal.

But, unfortunately, possibility 2 is very likely to happen as well. When a food object hits the voice box, it causes choking and coughing, but once it goes past the voice box, it will travel down the windpipe (which, at this age, is about the diameter and consistency of an oversized, jumbo drinking straw). At the end of the windpipe, there is a fork in the road, where there is a right side (leading to the right lung) and a left side (leading to the left lung). Very commonly, a foreign object will lodge on one side (most often the right, as the passage to the right lung is more of a straight angle than that to the left). When it lodges on one side, your baby can breathe comfortably from the

CHOKING EPISODES ARE ONE OF THE MOST COMMON HOUSEHOLD INJURIES IN CHILDREN

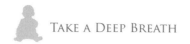

other side for a good period of time (anywhere from hours to WEEKS). But eventually, (in a matter of hours or weeks), your baby will start to show signs of distress. She may have more coughing, wheezing on the side where the object is lodged, or may seem to have **retractions** (where the neck, chest, and stomach muscles are pulling in and out during breathing). If she doesn't show signs of distress right away, she may develop what seems to be a respiratory illness like bronchitis or pneumonia in the weeks that follow. I once saw a little boy who was diagnosed with 'asthma' for months on end. No medicine was helping, so his parents sought another opinion from a new asthma doctor, who astutely noted that he was only wheezing from one side. Lo and behold, there was a crushed peanut lodged in his right lower windpipe. No asthma! So if you witness a choking event in your baby, even if she seems fine right afterwards, have her pediatrician take a look. Listening to the chest with a good pediatric stethoscope can elicit whether the lungs sound 'equally clear'. Sometimes your doctor will get an X-ray of the chest, to see if there is blockage of airflow in one lung. This can usually be seen if your baby lies on her side during the X-ray. If there is suspicion that the object is lodged, a specialist (either an ear, nose, and throat specialist or a pulmonary specialist) will place a camera down the baby's windpipe during a brief **general anesthesia** (meaning your baby needs to be completely asleep for this) and remove the object.

My seven-month old is perfectly healthy, but very often when she breathes in, it sounds like a squeak. She does this especially when she's playing.

Babies at this age are still developing coordination of breathing, making noise, and even laughing. Some part of what your baby is doing may be attributable to immature coordination of the airway reflexes. She means to make a noise but breathes in instead; she's so excited that she takes such a quick breath that her vocal cords come together, producing a squeaky sound. Babies are also deliberately experimenting with the sounds that they make. If they are excited, they may WANT to breathe in and shriek at the same time, producing what seems to be squeaky breathing. If she seems playful, is not struggling, and does not have retractions when she does this (and she didn't just choke on a carrot), then these are just normal noises that your baby is trying.

My 10-month-old has been teething, and was crying all night. He woke up this morning and his voice sounds very rough and weak. Can babies get laryngitis? Did he damage anything by all that crying?

Yes, babies can get laryngitis, and no, it is very unlikely that he did any damage to his voice box from all that crying. (This also goes for the crying of sleep training, if you are so inclined. Concerns for both psychological as well as physical damage from 'crying it out' have been shown to be unfounded in many studies). But your baby can develop some swelling in his voice box, and become hoarse from crying. Try not to let this add to your guilt of his pain (whether it be from teething or sleep training). The hoarseness is not particularly painful in and of itself. The best treatment is time (and ideally less crying), but you can also try increasing fluid intake, a humidifier in his bedroom, and reducing citrus or acidic foods for a few days. The hoarseness may linger for a week or more, but it should start to subside once the crying does.

My baby was born prematurely, and had a breathing tube in her throat for three months. She has a very weak cry. Will this get better?

Tiny babies, even extremely premature ones (born at 26 weeks or less, weighing as little as one pound), can handle having breathing tubes for very long periods of time. The care that babies receive in today's neonatal (newborn) intensive care units (NICU's) is extraordinary, and great efforts are taken to minimize irritation to the voice box or windpipe. However, if a tiny baby (or even a not-so-tiny baby) has a plastic tube in her air passage for any period of time, she is bound to develop some scar tissue. The tube acts as a chronic irritant just by being there. It also prevents the delicate linings of the voice box and windpipe from remaining smooth and mucus-lined. While the smallest tube possible is used (some almost as narrow as a cocktail straw), there is still bound to be some irritation. When the breathing tube does come out, the air passages, including the voice box, windpipe, and even lungs, will have some swelling. The swelling may heal into the scar tissue, leading to some roughness in her breathing or voice. Thankfully, most of the scarring goes away on its own, and children will have minimal voice problems as they get older.

The voice box itself can have some temporary damage, as the presence of the breathing tube makes the vocal cords pushed open (like an open 'V') for as long as the tube is in. In normal sound production of crying, the 'V' shape closes to make a

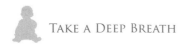

sound and opens when air goes through. This opening and closing works like a hinge on a door. If the hinge is stuck open, with no 'oil' or movement, that hinge will be a little stiff and creaky. Your baby may be hoarse from the stiffened 'hinge' on their voice box, so that when she tries to make a sound, it sounds weak or 'breathy'. Usually this improves with time, as the hinges become looser, in absence of the breathing tube. Your doctor may ask an ear, nose, and throat specialist to take a look to make sure that the vocal cords are moving well, and that there are no areas of irritation, swelling, or permanent scarring that need to be removed.

THE BIG PICTURE

Infants under one year continue to make unusual sounds from their throat. Occasionally these are purposeful, during play or laughter, but occasionally these are out of their control. While many of the noises babies make are not of any concern (except that they are noisy), some sounds are more worrisome. Around this age, the more concerning sounds are those that come on suddenly — either after a choking event, or during a respiratory illness. Most babies who have noisy breathing after the age of three months have already had some type of noisy breathing before then. If the sound suddenly changes, or if your baby seems to be suddenly struggling to breathe, these are times to get medical attention right away. More often than not, you may notice fluctuations in your baby's noisy breathing. It may be noisier during playtime, crawling, or early stages of walking. It may be noisier when she has a cold, or after crying. Voice problems are rare at this stage, but infants can still develop laryngitis from prolonged crying. It will go away relatively quickly, and needs almost no treatment.

DON'T WORRY

If your baby has already been diagnosed with a floppy throat (laryngomalacia), or is newly diagnosed in later infancy, expect some mild variations in the 'noisiness', depending on her activity. Most babies with this entity will have noisier breathing while eating, crying, and during some activity, and quieter breathing during rest and sleep. Expect there to be some increase in the noise until approximately the age of six to nine months, at which point things will begin to gradually improve. Most babies with laryngomalacia will have minimal to no noise by their first birthday, assuming it was mild or moderate to begin with.

Hoarseness in babies is rare but not dangerous. If it is from a crying episode (or episodes), it will subside in time. If the hoarseness is from having had a breathing tube, the timing of improvement depends on many factors — how long the breathing tube was in, how small your baby was, whether or not there are lung or heart issues, and whether or not there is stiffness of the 'hinges' in the voice box. A specialist's evaluation, where the doctor will place a tiny camera in your baby's nose or mouth to see her voice box, will give you a better sense of how long it will take for your baby's voice to strengthen.

WORRY

If your baby develops any kind of noisy breathing suddenly, call your doctor or seek medical attention right away. The possible explanations are numerous, and it is not up to you to have to figure them out. Some of the possible reasons may be:

❖   A choking episode (food, toy, seed)
❖   A respiratory illness leading to sudden swelling in the air passages
❖   A chronic throat problem that becomes exacerbated by an acute illness
❖   A lung problem, such as pneumonia, that may also cause inflammation in the throat.

In any event, I always say 'Don't worry alone'. This goes for parents, caregivers, and even doctors. When in doubt, call for help.

TO-DO LIST: THROATY NOISES AND STRIDOR

1. Look at your baby. If she is making noises, but is playing comfortably, sleeping well, and eating well, it is unlikely that there is something to worry about, unless it comes on suddenly.

2. If your baby had some noisy breathing as a young infant, chances are he may have some fluctuation in his breathing as he becomes more active.

3. It's ok to let your baby cry. She wont break anything (except maybe your sanity).

4. If you think your baby may have choked on something, even if he seems fine afterwards, seek medical attention right away.

Source for Throaty Noises in Babies:
www.pediatric-ent.com/learning/problems/hoarse

Chapter Ten

Feeding Issues
for Healthy Breathing

Sometime between ages four and six months, you will begin to feed your baby solid food. This is great fun! You break out the video cameras, and watch as your baby grabs the spoon, and gives you a look which seems to say 'what were you waiting for?' as she gobbles down the rice cereal/slurry. You call the relatives. You break out those cute pink bunny bowls you received as baby gifts, seemingly a lifetime ago. You hope that your baby will begin to sleep through the night (if she hasn't already), as you've increased her calorie intake a whopping fifty calories per day with all of that cereal. But cereal is just the beginning of this exciting adventure! There are mushy peas, mashy green beans, and smashy carrots to follow! And it gets better — teething crackers, food with texture, food with taste. So what does all of this have to do with breathing? Indeed, it has a lot to do with breathing. First of all, babies with **gastroesophageal reflux disease (GERD)** (see Chapter Three, Section One) may begin to show signs of improvement after solid food is started. Second of all (and the focus of this chapter), the start of solid food is one step closer to your baby's independence, and in turn, one step further away from you. But not to worry, this will not lessen the bond, loosen the string, or pull her away in any true sense. You will still be her source of food (until she can open the fridge in a year or two). You will still be able to choose what she eats, when she eats it, and how much she eats. But not for long! As babies get closer to their first birthday, they become more mobile, more dexterous, and develop better, quicker eye-hand coordination. That translated into baby speak is 'Me see that food on the floor. Me grab it quickly and put it in my mouth. Yum'. This independence needs to be closely monitored, and it

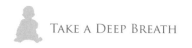

begins with your awareness about how your growing baby maneuvers food, what is and is not safe to give them, and why.

My baby has a floppy airway (laryngomalacia). She is six months old. Is it safe to start solid food?

It's always prudent to confirm with your doctor that your baby is ready to start solids. The American Academy of Pediatrics (AAP) recommends that babies begin solids at six months old. Part of this recommendation relates to their physical and motor coordination at this age, whereby babies are able to support their heads, move solid food to the back of their mouth with their tongues, and swallow solid textures into their esophagus. The other part of this recommendation has to do with breast-fed babies. Breast milk has very low iron content (formula has slightly more). By the age of six months, babies' stored iron from birth begins to be depleted, and needs to be replaced in their diet. Infant cereals such as rice cereal are fortified with iron, providing the supplementation babies need. Iron deficiency can lead to **anemia**, or low blood count. Babies with anemia may look pale, have overall weakness or low energy, and are more susceptible to infections.

Babies with floppy airways often have some choking with feeds of formula or breastmilk, but they usually do better with solid foods. This is because solids move more slowly, and allow for the tongue to push the food past the throat, towards the esophagus. It is not recommended that you give your baby, especially one with a challenging airway issue, rice cereal in their milk or formula as a drink in their bottle. It needs to be spooned in gradually, so they do not choke. In general, there is no reason why your baby should not start solids at the age of six months, even if she has a floppy airway. That said, if your baby has had severe feeding difficulties, she might need to have a swallowing evaluation before beginning solid foods. Your pediatrician can determine if this is necessary, and can refer you to a speech/swallow specialist (speech pathologists with specific training in evaluating and treating infants and children with swallowing issues) for

AFTER AGE SIX MONTHS, BABIES NEED IRON IN THEIR DIETS

an evaluation. These specialist evaluations usually include having the therapist watch your baby drink and eat, followed by a series of video-X-rays performed while your baby is drinking or eating different consistencies. These videos will enable the therapist to determine which food textures are best for your baby.

My six-month-old is getting tired of the different types of infant cereals. Is there an order of foods I should give him?

Many pediatricians, nutritionists, and parents are firm believers in proceeding in a very specific order of food types when introducing new foods to a baby. The idea is to start with all of those nasty green vegetables that children notoriously hate, then give them a treat with the golden sweet potatoes and carrots, followed by the icing on the cake — pureed fruit in a jar. In reality, the most important point is to try one food at a time (either one new food per day, or one new food per meal). The main reason for this is to make sure that your baby does not have an allergic reaction to a new food. These allergies may not appear right away. Some will appear as a rash on the face; others may present as gassy bloating, diarrhea, or even a ring-like diaper rash the next day. Aside from monitoring for allergies, the order of food introduction is really up to you. Some kids really do like green beans or peas. And some don't like peaches — no matter when you started them. And the old tenet still holds — if he refuses, try it again. And again. Three tries per food, at least. And it may not be the food itself, but the way it's prepared, or the particular brand. One thing is for sure — if you cook frozen peas and then put them in the blender yourself, they taste ten thousand times better than the jarred ones. Root vegetables, such as carrots and potatoes, should not be cooked fresh for your baby, as they may contain too many nitrates. It's best to use the store-bought jars for these, as the manufacturers will remove nitrates found in the soil of these foods. These nitrate levels are a concern only in the first months of your baby's solids. As your baby approaches his first birthday, it is fine to make these fresh as well.

When can I give my baby REAL solid food, and not just the pureed baby food?

'Real' solid food should be introduced gradually. One way to do this is to feed your baby food that you grind or blend yourself. That way, you can create the consistency

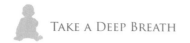

that works best for your baby. Usually at about nine months, babies can handle pureed food that has very soft pieces of cooked pasta, rice, or vegetables. Give your baby time with these. It may take a bit longer for her to negotiate the larger pieces around her tongue, past her throat, and into her esophagus. While it may have become second nature for her to take larger and larger spoons full of pureed foods, the larger chunks should be given in smaller amounts, with breaks in between each spoonful to make sure she hasn't held any in the back of her mouth before swallowing. While many of the baby food jars are labeled 'Nine months and up', remember that this is just a guideline, and that many babies are not ready for such foods at nine, or even ten months. Do not be frustrated if your baby is that baby. If she still is better able to handle fully pureed foods, then so it is. Even if the nine-month-old geniuses around her are chewing on steak, and eating with a fork and knife, your child will not be banished to poor school performance or low self-esteem if she is still just being a baby, eating baby food. Don't rush this. Self-regulation is an underrated skill at this age. Let her take what she can handle. She will progress at her pace, and be all the smarter for it.

When feeding your baby solid food, especially if it is a new consistency, make sure that you are in the room and facing her. While this may seem obvious to you at first, once she starts to self-feed (at about nine months, that magic *average* age, babies have better ability to grab solid objects and put them in their own mouth), you may be more inclined to pop out of the room to answer the phone, check your email, or even (heaven forbid) take a shower. But just because your baby is securely strapped into her high chair does not mean that she is necessarily safe from having a choking accident on food. Even if it is a food she has eaten comfortably before, always be in the room with your baby when she is eating.

My baby can now hold his own bottle, and feed himself his formula. Can he drink this in the car? What about finger food snacks?
I don't recommend this, unless there is an adult sitting with him in the back seat. Until the age two years, infants and children should be in a rear — facing seat in the back seat of your car. While you may have rigged a rearview mirror attachment

so that you can see your baby's face at any time you choose, you really should have your eyes on the road. While it is extremely unlikely that a baby at an age where they can hold their own bottle will choke on the liquid, it is certainly possible that they can, and you may not see or hear it happen. Finger food snacks are a definite no-no in the car, especially in a rear – facing car seat (and even afterwards). You may have to stop suddenly while in traffic, and this may lead your baby (or even older child) to choke on whatever he's eating or drinking. Choking events while eating solids in the car are not as rare as you'd think. While the idea of silence and contentment is great, especially if you are stuck in traffic with a cranky baby, safety in the car is critical.

INFANTS SHOULD BE IN REAR-FACING CAR SEATS UNTIL THE AGE OF TWO YEARS

My ten-month old only has two teeth. How will he be able to chew any food?

Timing of tooth eruption in babies is variable, with a wide range of what is considered to be 'normal'. On average, babies get their first two teeth (the bottom center ones – lower central incisors) between the age of six and eight months, followed by the top two (upper central incisors). In general, they continue to alternate between bottom and top after that. Most babies do not have molars or premolars before the age of 12 months, but they are still able to 'chew' soft food. The front teeth have relatively little to do with chewing the food, so don't be concerned about absence of teeth in relation to soft solid foods. Even with no teeth, babies can eat food that has the consistency of overcooked pasta or rice. Most of the mashing comes from the back part of the gums, and the food gets moved from the front to the back by the muscles of the tongue and cheeks. Babies without teeth can even 'chew' (or gnaw) on very hard teething crackers (the harder the cracker, the less likely it will break apart into unsafe large chunks in their mouth). Teething can take months, and those crackers are soothing, especially when frozen. But again, don't give your baby a teething cracker in the car.

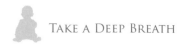
What about giving my 11-month food that is crunchy, like crackers or bread?

Every child is different in his or her timing of being able to eat various consistencies and types of foods. Certain foods are not recommended in children under one year because of risks of infection. For instance, honey is not recommended under one year because of the risk of '**infant botulism**', an illness affecting your baby's nervous system due to a toxin found in honey that affects only young infants. This is the same 'toxin' seen in Botox®, which smoothes our aging faces by temporarily paralyzing the muscles that cause wrinkles. This just goes to show you that one baby's toxin is another parent's treat.

As far as breathing risks, the most important safety measure you can take is to be with your baby face-to-face when trying new foods, and to make sure that your baby is secured in a highchair or booster seat. Always err on the side of overcooking foods such as vegetables, meats, and even fruits. Start with tiny pieces, the size of your pinky fingernail, to see how she handles it in her mouth. Babies love crusty bread, especially if they are teething, but be careful of some of the large dry crusts of French bread, or even the doughy center of bagels. They may get too much in their little mouths at once, and choke on it. Soft crackers and bread are great for babies, and dry cereal such as Cheerios® can also be introduced before her first birthday.

What foods should I absolutely avoid before age one?

While the Consumer Product Safety Commission (CPSC) has mandated that all children's toys be labeled with safety guidelines based on age, there are no such guidelines for food safety. You may notice that *some* foods are labeled for safety precautions (some hotdogs, and some baby/toddler foods), but there are no national guidelines in order to date. However, here is a list of some foods that are absolutely NOT recommended to give to babies under 12 months:

❖ Nuts or seeds of any kind
❖ Candy of any kind, including gum and lollipops
❖ Popcorn
❖ Hotdogs

* Raw vegetables
* Raw fruit with skins
* Grapes (unless peeled and cut into tiny pieces)
* Raisins (or any dried fruit)
* Peanut butter (or any nut butter)

What are some healthy, safe food choices for my baby under 12 months?

There are many foods that young infants can enjoy, once they have mastered and are ready to move beyond pureed baby food. Some great options include:

* Well — cooked meat, chicken, or fish, cut into tiny pieces
* Well — cooked vegetables of any kind, cut into tiny pieces
* Peeled soft fruits, such as plums, peaches, pears, bananas, or grapes, cut into tiny pieces
* Berries — blueberries, raspberries, blackberries, strawberries
* Cooked hard fruits (peels removed), such as apples, cut into tiny pieces
* Sliced avocado
* Yogurt
* Bread
* Soft crackers, or really hard teething crackers
* Rice
* Pasta
* Couscous
* Cheese cut into thin slices (not cubes)

When making 'real' food, you should do so without any seasoning. Salt or pepper is not necessary for young babies. While these are not dangerous, babies need to be able to taste actual food, and need not rely on added spices to enjoy what they eat.

What do I do if my baby chokes on a piece of food?

It's wise for all parents and caregivers to receive training in infant and child **cardiopulmonary resuscitation (CPR)**. These courses are given at most local community hospitals on a regular basis, or at adult education centers, schools, or a local

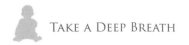

Red Cross (www.redcross.org). Many hospitals will offer CPR training during pregnancy or if you are planning to adopt a baby. But even the most trained, prepared parent is not really expecting to use this training. Food choking events in children are one of the most common household injuries, and account for over 10,000 emergency room visits per year in the United States alone. *One child dies every five days from a choking event in this country.* While many choking events occur unwitnessed (a crawling baby finds something interesting such as a lone peanut or a whole coffee bean on the kitchen floor), there are life-saving measures you should know.

If you see your baby choking but do not see the object, do not stick your finger in her mouth. That will make her choke more, and very likely push the object further into her air passage.

What are the steps I need to know to save my baby if she chokes?

Nobody ever wants to be in the position to save a baby, but if the situation does arise, there are critical steps one should know. It's good to get in the habit of reviewing these as your baby grows — every six months until she is three years old, and every year after that. Call your local Red Cross to see where you and any of your child's caregivers can receive training. Many of these training programs are offered in multiple languages.

1. If your baby chokes, she may cough, gag, or cry. If she is coughing or crying, her airway is not completely blocked. Let her continue to cough. She may be able to dislodge the object on her own.
2. If she is suddenly unable to cough or cry, and she cannot make any sound, her airway is completely blocked. You may notice her skin turn bright red or blue.
3. Ask someone to call 911 right away. If you are alone, attend to your baby for two minutes, and then call 911.
4. If there is complete airway blockage (no noise from your baby), and you think she choked on something, try to dislodge the object. Hold her, face down, on your arm or thigh, making sure her head is lower than the rest of her body. Using the heel of your hand, give five firm back blows between her shoulder blades to help force the object out of her throat.

5. If back blows are not successful, carefully turn your baby's face upwards, supporting her head with one hand. Place three fingers at the center point between her nipples, and give five chest thrusts, pushing down ½ to 1 inch, approximately 1 to 2 seconds apart.
6. Continue this sequence of back blows and chest thrusts until your baby begins to cough.
7. If she becomes unconscious, you will need to begin CPR.

How do I administer CPR?

If your baby has choked, and you are unable to dislodge the object, have someone call 911 and begin CPR. If you are by yourself, give two minutes of CPR, then call 911 and continue CPR. By giving CPR, you are administering oxygen to your baby's blood by your own breath, and are aiding circulation of her blood by giving chest compressions.

1. If your baby is not coughing or breathing after attempt at dislodging the object, give two breaths. To do this, have your baby lying flat, on a firm surface. Tilt her neck back gently, and lift her chin slightly. Put your mouth over your baby's nose and mouth and give two little breaths.* Remember, your baby's lungs are much smaller than yours, and you do not need to give large breaths.
2. If there is no breathing, give thirty chest compressions, using the tips of two or three of your fingers just below the midpoint of her nipples. Each chest compression should compress about ½ to 1 inch down into the chest. Give one to two compressions every second (approximately 100 times per minute).
3. Continue this cycle of two breaths/30 compressions until help comes.
4. Before giving a breath cycle, check your baby's mouth to see if you can see the dislodged object. If you can fully see it, you can grab it out of her mouth.

---

*According to the American Heart Association, it is now recommended that CPR for adults begin with chest compressions, not breathing support. But because infants and children are more likely to have an airway event as opposed to a cardiac event leading to an emergency with no breathing or heartbeat, the baby's airway can be addressed first.

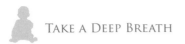
WHEN YOU CALL 911, TRY TO STAY CALM!
IT WILL BE IMPOSSIBLE TO STAY CALM! BUT TRY TO SPEAK CLEARLY AND LISTEN TO THE OPERATOR'S INSTRUCTIONS.
TRY TO DESCRIBE WHAT HAPPENED TO YOUR BABY AND WHAT IS HAPPENING AT THE TIME YOU CALL.
GIVE YOUR LOCATION AND PHONE NUMBER.
FOLLOW THE 911 OPERATOR'S INSTRUCTIONS ON WHAT TO DO.
DO NOT HANG UP UNTIL THE 911 OPERATOR TELLS YOU TO.

THE BIG PICTURE

When it comes to your baby's first solids, the most important safety measure is that you are watching him eat. At first, this will be easy and obvious, as he will need to be fed spoonfuls of pureed food. But as he gets more independent, and gains interests in different foods and textures, you will need to be more vigilant regarding what goes in his mouth. Always have him seated securely during mealtime. Be as careful as you can when preparing your own meals or meals for older children in your family. When cutting vegetables, for instance, it's easy to have a carrot slice fall on the floor. Find it, because you don't want it to end up in the mouth of a crawling infant. Some families play it extra safe, and keep all potentially dangerous foods out of the house, such as nuts, candy, and popcorn. If nothing else, keep them out of reach of ALL children. That way, you can be physically present and aware if an older child is having a snack with these types of foods. Educate older children and adult caregivers regarding food safety and choking risks. Avoid unnecessary distractions for older children, such as toys or running around during meal or snack times. Various cultures and generations have differing ideas on safety in this area. Make sure you are all on the same page (*your* page).

At about nine months, babies usually advance their diet from pureed baby food to soft solid foods, such as pasta, rice, and soft fruits such as bananas. Always start slowly when introducing new foods and textures, and start with small amounts in tiny pieces. If your baby seems to gag on something, even if it's soft, give her some time to cough or swallow it herself. If she seems to continue to do this each time she tries this food, take a step back instead of forging ahead. She will get it in her own time. Babies without teeth are still able to eat and 'chew' solid foods. However, babies do not develop molars and premolars (the molar — like teeth just in front of the molars) until after the first birthday, so avoid foods that need to be ground up in the mouth, such as raw fruits, raw vegetables, or nuts. When in doubt, check with your pediatrician on which food is, or is not, safe to give your baby.

DON'T WORRY

Every baby is different in his or her progression from a full liquid diet of formula or breast milk to solid food. Some welcome solids with an 'it's about time' look in their eyes, and some prefer to continue as is, with the comfort of the bottle or breast. And most babies will fluctuate in their interests. She may begin by absolutely loving the solids, even the mushy rice cereal. He may plow through the rainbow of green, yellow, and orange vegetables, and reject the sweet fruit (although this is highly unlikely). What's more common is that she may, at some point into the food progression, reject food altogether, and accept only milk or formula again. She obviously didn't read the instruction book! But don't be too frustrated. Babies are excellent at self-regulation when it comes to intake. If he is hungry enough, he will eat something at some point. You may need to limit the amount of liquids he gets in order to do this, but don't get too caught up in the exact amounts of each, as long as he is taking in small amounts of solids.

When it comes to more 'solid' solid food, err on the side of soft and small. This will be a learning experience for you and your baby. There is no rush, and he will figure it out. Give him options, but keep an eye on him at all times.

WORRY

If your baby absolutely refuses to take in solids such as rice cereal, he may have a swallowing disorder that needs to be addressed by your pediatrician, who may refer you to a speech and swallow specialist. If your baby develops severe cramping, diarrhea, or a rash after trying a new food, it may be a food allergy. Discontinue the food of concern, and give your doctor a call.

If your baby has a choking episode while eating (or you think he may have choked on food), begin emergency treatment as outlined in this chapter. No parent or caregiver ever wishes to have to use these measures, but knowledge and caution can save a baby's life.

TO-DO LIST: FEEDING ISSUES FOR HEALTHY BREATHING

1. Feeding solids to your baby is fun! Enjoy this!

2. Be patient with your baby's dietary changes. Expect some ups and downs when your baby's diet expands. Likes and dislikes will fluctuate. Give breaks, try things again, and be positive. Your baby will pick up on any anxiety or concerns that you have.

3. Keep unsafe foods out of reach of your baby, especially when he starts crawling or walking.

4. Make sure that all who have contact with your baby (including any older children) are aware of choking risks with certain food types. Be firm, especially with relatives or other caregivers who may have different ideas on food safety.

5. Take an infant CPR class at your local Red Cross or hospital. If you did this before your baby was born, it's always good to take refresher courses. Make sure any caregiver has this training as well. Many centers offer CPR courses in more than one language.

6. Local hospitals, Red Cross chapters, and even pediatricians' offices offer small posters with CPR instructions and illustrations. Post one of these on an easily visible wall in your kitchen.

7. Do not give your baby snacks while you are driving (this includes lollypops). Even if he is a comfortable eater, you may need to stop or turn suddenly, leading him to choke.

8. If you are unsure whether or not a new food is safe to feed your baby, check with your doctor first.

Sources for Feeding Safety in Babies:

www.redcross.org

www.babycenter.com

www.fedhealth.net

www.entnet.org/healthinformation/choking-campaign.cfm

Liebsch B, Leibsch J. It's a Disaster! A Disaster Preparedness, Prevention, and Basic
    First Aid Manual. Fedhealth. 2006

Chapter Eleven

Sleepy Breathing in the First Year

Hopefully sometime before the first birthday, your baby will begin to sleep through the night. You may have established a cozy, quiet bedtime ritual, whether it's a bath, a story, a song, or a cuddle. You've learned to put your baby down while she is awake but sleepy, and now she is able to doze off on her own. You close her door, congratulate yourself, and maybe even enjoy a quiet dinner with your spouse, have a glass of wine, watch TV, read the newspaper for the first time since pregnancy, or just relax and close your eyes. You turn on the baby monitor, sit down, put your feet up, and — what's that noise?? Is that my beautiful angel I hear? Is she snoring? I thought I heard normal breathing, but then I heard nothing for a few seconds, and then a gasp. What happened to my newly found evenings of quiet time and rest?

At the end of the first year, some babies begin to snore or make strange noises during sleep. For the most part, these are of no concern, especially if your baby remains asleep and comfortable through the night. There are, however, some changes that may develop in your baby's nose and mouth that may need to be addressed, especially if these noises are associated with your baby waking up several times at night.

My ten-month-old naps twice per day, and has been sleeping through the night for the last three months. Over the last few weeks, it sounds like he's snoring. Is this possible? I thought it was only a problem of older, overweight men.

Snoring in infants and children was previously unrecognized or dismissed as 'normal', but it has been increasingly understood and studied as being on the spectrum of

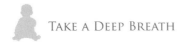

sleep disorders, or more commonly known as **Obstructive sleep apnea (OSA)**. Obstructive sleep apnea is a period during sleep where a person makes effort to breathe for at least two breath cycles, but despite this effort, there is no air movement. In an adult, who breathes about 12 times per minute during sleep, this means that there is no air movement for at least ten seconds. An infant or young child breathes about 20 times per minute during sleep, so 'apnea' (no breathing) occurs if there is no air movement (during effort of breathing) for at least five or six seconds. This needs to be differentiated from **central sleep apnea**, which is very commonly seen in younger infants. Central sleep apnea occurs because very young infants, under the age of three months, have immature brain regulation of breathing. The part of the brain that 'tells' the baby to breathe is not fully developed, and it is very common for healthy babies to have periods of 'central apnea' during sleep, lasting six to ten seconds. These episodes are normal. A baby with central apnea is not making an effort to breathe, then breathes regularly for a period of time, and then may repeat this cycle. Most parents don't even know that their baby has these events, as they are not distressing to the baby, and are silent. Babies grow out of central apnea in the first three months. Rarely, there are babies who have severe central apnea, where they stop breathing for so long that they develop a blue discoloration, or **cyanosis**, during seemingly effortless periods of central sleep apnea. This is an issue that needs to be addressed with your pediatrician. It is extremely rare, and is usually seen in babies with other medical problems of the heart, lung, or brain, but if you notice any color change when your baby is sleeping, call your doctor right away.

While snoring in itself is not sleep apnea, it is on the spectrum of it. The noise of snoring is because there is some sort of blockage in the air passages, either in the nose, the back of the nose, or the mouth. If the breathing pattern is 'regular', where it sounds like there is a steady (albeit noisy) beat, it is not OSA, but just snoring. But if you hear snoring, followed by a pause in breathing, followed by a gasp, then that is more on the end of the spectrum towards OSA.

If you hear your baby starting to snore, check to see what's going on when the noise occurs. If it came on all of a sudden, it may be that your baby simply has a stuffy nose or a cold. You may want to try to position your baby on his side, or spray his nose with saline. If he does not seem to have a cold, you may want to see if it's happening on a regular basis. If so, let your pediatrician know. It may be a sign of an environmental allergy, or enlarged **tonsils** or **adenoids.**

What are tonsils and adenoids? Can they be an issue in the first year of life?

Tonsils and **adenoids** are **lymph nodes** (little round growths that are part of our immune system) that are located inside our mouth. We have thousands of lymph nodes in our body, and hundreds in our neck and throat alone. The tonsils are two lymph nodes located at the back of the mouth, one on each side. They look like small, pink, sponge-like structures. Most babies younger than two years old have very tiny, barely visible tonsils, and it is extremely rare (although not impossible) for babies in the first year of life to have enlarged tonsils. In fifteen years of practicing pediatric ear, nose, and throat surgery in a busy academic urban medical center, I have seen only two children under the age of one year who have had enlarged tonsils to the degree of causing snoring and breathing problems. The reason for this rarity is that the tonsils, adenoids, and other lymph nodes tend to undergo a period of growth between ages two and six years. It rarely occurs before this. The adenoids (plural, but they are actually one 'area' of lymph node tissue) are located way in the back of the nose, up behind the roof of the mouth. We cannot see adenoids unless we place a tiny camera the diameter of a spaghetti strand into the back of the nose. When the adenoids are enlarged, they can cause nasal congestion and snoring. As with tonsils, they usually don't become an area of concern until after the age of two years, but adenoid enlargement is more common than tonsil enlargement in infants.

BREATHING DURING SLEEP SHOULD BE SILENT

If you think your baby is snoring, and may have a tonsil or adenoid issue, have your pediatrician take a look. Most will recommend watchful waiting, assuming that the snoring issue is not a major interference with your baby's sleep quality.

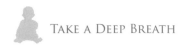

I'm not sure if my baby has 'normal' sleep. I think she may have sleep apnea, but I'm not sure. Some nights it sounds like she's just snoring, but some nights she really seems to be struggling to breathe during sleep. Is there a way of figuring this out?

Sometimes your doctor will ask you to make a quick video or audio tape of your baby's sleep, to get a better sense of what your baby's breathing pattern is. By hearing or seeing this, your doctor may be able to give you tips on position changes, such as having your baby sleep on her side or keeping the head of her bed a bit elevated with a crib wedge or a small pillow. If it seems as if your baby is really struggling, she may recommend that your baby have a **sleep study** (technically called a **polysomnogram**). These non-invasive tests are performed in sleep laboratories, and are most accurately performed if done on an overnight basis, as opposed to during one of your child's daytime naps. Your baby will come in during the evening (with you, of course), and a sleep technician will attach monitors to measure her oxygen levels, breathing rate, breathing patterns, and muscle movements. A trained sleep specialist (either a neurologist, pulmonologist, or ear, nose and throat specialist), will interpret the measurements of your baby's breathing from the overnight test, and determine whether or not there is a sleep disorder such as sleep apnea. Some sleep study companies will be able to do 'mini' sleep studies in your home. The obvious benefit of the at-home studies is that your baby and you are in the comfort of your own home. The main downsides are that they often times don't provide as much information, and many insurance providers will not cover the costs of the at-home studies. The main point of the sleep study is to determine whether or not your baby has a breathing pattern that is on the spectrum of sleep apnea, or one that is on the spectrum of just noisy snoring. If you and your pediatrician are unsure by just listening to or watching your baby, it's always best to get a sleep study. It is not invasive (there are no probes or needles, and no medication is needed), but most babies (and even older children and adults) dislike the sticky monitors that are placed on their body for the study. Some babies (and older children and adults) will rip off the monitors in the middle of the night. Sometimes these monitors can be replaced, but some babies will have no part of it. To have the best chance of a successful (meaning completed) sleep study, make sure that the sleep center or home sleep study company is one that works with infants and children on a regular basis.

Assuming that a sleep study is successfully completed, your child will receive a 'score', called an **Apnea/Hypopnea Index (AHI).** This score is a measurement of how many 'events' (either loud snoring or complete apnea) occur on average in an hour during sleep. It will be noted on the sleep study (especially if performed in a sleep laboratory) at what stages of sleep (lighter stages, deeper stages, dream stages) these events occur, and whether or not the baby's oxygen level in her blood drops during these events. Normal blood oxygen levels in both children and adults is in the 95-100% range. A normal AHI score for a sleep study is zero events of obstruction per hour. An AHI of 1 or higher is considered abnormal in children, and an AHI of 5 or higher is considered abnormal in adults. That said, if your baby has a mildly elevated AHI (1 to 5), but has normal oxygen levels, it is in all likelihood a very mild degree of sleep apnea that needs to be monitored by your doctor. She may want to repeat the sleep study in six to twelve months. A very high AHI, certainly anything greater than ten, with episodes of low oxygen, may merit a visit to a specialist — either pulmonary (lung) or ear, nose, and throat, to better assess if and where a blockage in the baby's airway is leading to breathing issues with sleep.

My eight-month-old sounds 'gurgly' and congested at night. Is there anything this can be besides big tonsils or adenoids?

Of course — but now I'll ask you a question. Are you giving him a bottle of milk or formula in his bed? While this may be an absolutely heavenly way for your baby (and therefore you) to go off to sleep peacefully, the milk or formula may lead to several concerning issues. Besides contributing to tooth/gum decay and minimizing your baby's ability to self-soothe, a bottle of anything but water in the crib can contribute to breathing problems, including snoring and sleep apnea. There are several reasons for this: (1) the milk/formula itself is somewhat thick in consistency, and can mix with your baby's saliva and mucus, creating a gummy mass of goo at the back of her throat; (2) milk/formula consumption may actually cause some increase in mucus production, leading to more congestion; (3) when falling off to sleep, (or even worse, during sleep), the muscles of the throat, neck, esophagus and stomach become very relaxed, making the movement of milk down the digestive tract slower, leading to even more liquid being pooled in the throat and mouth; (4) drinking (even water, for that matter) while lying flat will most definitely lead to some degree of **gastroesophageal reflux (GER).**

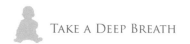

Not only will the milk move in the wrong direction, but the acid and fluids produced by the stomach lining may also move 'up' instead of down. The acid and fluid from the stomach may 'reflux' (go in the wrong direction) as high as the back of the nose, especially in babies. This can cause nasal congestion and swelling both during sleep as well as during wake hours. If your baby absolutely loves her night time feed (who wouldn't), I suggest creating a bedtime ritual of a bottle (or breastfeed) when upright, then some holding and cuddling (also upright), followed by putting her down. I know, easy for me to say, especially when I cant hear your baby screaming right now. But her bottle in the bed is just another habit/ritual that needs to be changed. It won't be easy. There are no magic answers, but whatever technique you choose (crying it out, gradual weaning by cutting the amount, switching to water, or even teaming up with your child to make a sleep 'plan' together), it will eventually work if you stick to your plan. Keep reminding yourself of that. There are very few (although not zero) five year olds who take a bottle to bed at night. Somehow they all stop at some point, but it will very likely not be their decision when it happens.

My baby snores. He doesn't have big tonsils or adenoids, and does not take a bottle to bed. What else could it be?

Another common reason for snoring in babies in their first year is allergies — not necessarily food allergies, but environmental allergies such as dust, pets, and pollen. Even if your baby is too young to be accurately tested for allergies, 'allergic response' to certain triggers may begin in the first year. Some babies with environmental allergies have no symptoms during the day, but are quite stuffy at night, and even during naptime. If your baby is snoring due to allergies, you may notice that he breathes comfortably during sleep if his mouth is open, but sounds very noisy when his mouth is closed. "Mouth-breathing" is usually a sign of nasal blockage, and allergies are certainly a good possible cause. If there are other family members with allergies, you may want to look into possible triggers that make your baby's nose stuffier. If there is carpeting in his room, you will need to clean it religiously, or even remove it. Parents are always amazed at how much dust collects on a bare floor on a regular basis. That same amount of dust was sitting in the carpet unnoticed. You may also have to experiment with different types of bedding, to see if that triggers allergic symptoms. If changes in your baby's environment don't help, you may want to ask your pediatrician about having your baby tested for allergies, at least to get a general sense of your baby's allergic tendencies (see Section Two, Chapter Eight). Unfortunately, there are virtually no allergy medications that are safe for babies under the age of one year, but if you know the allergens that cause the symptoms, you will be able to remove them. Saline nasal spray is useful for nasal allergies as well. There is no limit to the frequency that you can use nasal saline for your baby. A good way to remember to use it is to do so before naps and bedtime. When you use saline as a flush, where you insert the nozzle into your baby's nose, and give the bottle a good squeeze, it actually works to remove a large percentage of allergens from the nasal passages, along with the blocked mucus. If your baby has bad indoor allergies, you may consider purchasing an air purifier for his room. These remove tiny particles from the air, minimizing the irritants causing nasal stuffiness.

THE BIG PICTURE

It is not uncommon for babies to have occasional snoring, even before their first birthday. There are a few things you need to look for as they sleep. If you hear noise, but her breathing pattern is 'regular' (meaning there is a constant beat to it, without pauses or breaks) she likely has a mild degree of snoring, which does not need any further care or concern. But if you hear your baby snore very loudly (you can hear him in the next room, even without the baby monitor), or you notice that your baby's snores are intermixed with pauses in his breathing, followed by gasps for air, he may have a more significant sleep problem such as sleep apnea. If you notice that your baby has periods where he is trying to breathe (you see his chest or stomach muscles moving up and down) but there is no air movement, these are likely periods of apnea (no air movement). Try to record these episodes, either by audio or video, to show your pediatrician.

By the time your baby is able to hold a bottle on her own, you should think about minimizing and then eventually avoiding the bottle in the bed, during both naps and night time sleep. The reasons for this include both developmental (your baby needs to learn to self-soothe and put herself to sleep), and physical (the milk consumption while lying flat can contribute to snoring, nasal congestion, dental decay, and gastroesophageal reflux).

DON'T WORRY

Almost all children snore at some point. Some do so because they have a cold, mild allergies, or mild enlargement of their adenoids or tonsils. Some children will have none of these issues, but may snore especially during deep sleep, when the muscles at the back of the throat are extremely relaxed, so much so that these muscles hit up against each other and make a funny sound. Some may snore more when they are on their backs, but are quiet sleepers on their sides or stomachs. Mild variations in breathing patterns during a baby's sleep are normal, and if your baby is comfortable throughout the night, it is nothing to be concerned about. Mention it to your pediatrician at your child's next visit, and he may have some tips that are particular to your baby.

WORRY

If you think that your baby is really struggling to breathe at night, and you hear loud snoring with pauses in her breathing, she may have a degree of obstructive sleep apnea. There are multiple possible causes for this, but you should let your doctor know how often this is happening, and for how long. Snoring and sleep apnea is more common in older children (most commonly seen in age two- to six-year-olds), but it can certainly begin in the first year.

TO-DO LIST: SLEEPY BREATHING IN THE FIRST YEAR

1. Once your baby starts sleeping independently, check on her breathing. You may be surprised to hear some snoring.

2. If your baby does snore, do not worry, but check again at different times of night.

3. Try different sleep positions for your baby. Most babies with snoring sleep more comfortably on their sides or stomachs.

4. Do not put your baby on her stomach to sleep until she is old enough to roll onto her back independently during both wake time and sleep time. This usually occurs sometime between ages four and eight months.

5. If you think your baby snores very loudly, and you notice that he has some pauses in his breathing, followed by gasps for air, he may have sleep apnea. Make a brief audio or video tape, and bring it (and your baby) to your doctor.

6. Don't put your baby down to sleep with a bottle of breast milk or formula.

7. Pacifiers have no negative impact on sleep issues, and have even been found to reduce likelihood of SIDS. If a pacifier helps your baby stay asleep, keep a few in his crib, so he can grab an extra one if he spits it out.

8. If your baby seems stuffy at night, and there are other family members with allergies, she may be developing allergies as well. While there are no medications to give at this age, there are environmental changes you can make, and an air purifier may help as well.

Source for Sleepy Breathing in the First Year:

www.entnet.org/healthinformation/could-child-have-sleep-apnea

Chapter Twelve

Respiratory Illnesses in Babies: Croup and Crud

As your baby gets older, he will get more colds. Usually these are mild (albeit frequent), and the older he gets, the better he is at fighting them off more quickly. The reasons for the increase in colds with age are: (1) older babies tend to be 'out' more — with more exposure in public places, and more exposure to other babies, in either a day-care or a baby group. (2) the protective immunity that a baby has from his mother begins to fade after the first few months of life. Breast milk does contain some protective antibodies against illnesses, but the majority of these were acquired before birth. Sometimes a cold will turn into something completely different — not a sinus infection, throat infection, or fever, but something called **croup**. At least 15% of children will suffer from at least one episode of croup before the age of five years. Any parent who has had a child with croup can recognize it a mile away, but for a first-timer, it can be terrifying. The technical term for croup is **laryngotracheobron-chitis (LTB)**, and it is a sudden swelling of the upper airways. It usually occurs following a very mild cold (it is caused by a virus similar to the cold virus), and, as with most bad things, it occurs suddenly in the middle of the night. Croup occurs most commonly in the six-month to three-year-old age group, so you may see this occur before age one.

A rare, potentially life-threatening airway infection of this age group is thank-fully becoming a disease for the medical history books. This entity, called **epiglot-titis**, is a sudden swelling of the **epiglottis**, the floppy leaf-like flap that closes the air passage during eating and opens during breathing or talking. When the epiglot-tis swells in a child, it can completely block off the breathing passages in a matter

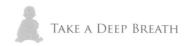

of hours. The epiglottis is most susceptible to infection by a bacteria called **Hemophilus influenzae (H. flu)**. This is not the 'flu' virus, but a very aggressive bacteria that can cause life-threatening illnesses such as epiglottitis or **meningitis** (infection of the fluid that surrounds the brain and spinal cord). When immunization against H. flu became standardized (the 'HiB' vaccine, the first dose of which is administered at the age of two months) epiglottitis and H. flu meningitis became nearly completely eradicated in the United States. After over a decade of working with children, I have never seen a case of epiglottitis in a child. Prior to the 1990's, many children would die every year from this infection.

My 11-month-old has had a runny nose, but no fever and seems to be acting fine. Right before putting her down to sleep, I noticed that she has this dry, brassy cough. What can I expect?

If your child is beginning to develop 'croup', you may be lucky enough to get a hint of it before you put her to sleep at night. However, the 'classic' presentation of croup is a baby who wakes in the middle of the night with a brassy/barky cough, sometimes accompanied by breathing trouble or '**stridor**' (you will hear a high-pitched squeak when your baby breathes in). Croup usually follows a mild cold, and often comes on suddenly. What's happening is that the very top part of the windpipe (below the voice box) becomes swollen, which causes some narrowing of the air passage, and leads to a dry, brassy cough. If you've heard a croup cough once, you will know it forever more. Next time you're at the zoo, listen to the barking seals. That's what croup sounds like.

If your baby is having croup for the first time, don't panic. But if she is experiencing a barking cough and also seems to be having trouble breathing (noisy breathing when she breathes in, chest or neck muscles pulling in, or has any blue discoloration to the skin), call 911. In most babies with a croupy cough, it is not quite that severe, and there is much you can do at home to remedy the symptoms. The best home remedy for croup is humidity. Pick up your baby (she will be more comfortable upright), and if you don't live in a desert, bring her outside in the cool night air. Croup season is usually the fall and spring, so it will probably be a bit cool outside. If it's wintry cold, bundle your baby in winter outer clothes, especially her head and feet (hat/boots, etc), and bring her outside. Rain is ideal (it's 100% humidity, after all), but keep her under an awning or bring an umbrella. If it's not cool, it may at least be humid, and humidity is the best home remedy for croup. You can also try turning on your shower all the way up on hot, closing the bathroom doors, and getting the bathroom very steamy. This often helps as well, even if the steam is warmer. Just don't put your baby in the hot shower. She does not need to get wet, nor does she need to burn herself. It is also a good time to break out the humidifier (or buy one in the morning, if you don't have one). If she seems better after a few minutes of outdoor or bathroom humidity, you can put her back to bed, with a humidifier on if you have one. Most babies who have a croupy night will be fine the next morning. You will be exhausted, but her cough will have remarkably subsided, until the next night. Most kids who have croup are fine, with minimal cough during the day. It's primarily a nocturnal illness. This is likely due to the fact that your baby is lying down, there is less humidity, and she is not able to clear her throat as effectively as when she's awake.

What if my baby is still coughing and seems uncomfortable after I try humidification at home?

If your baby is still sounding really noisy (barky cough, and seems to be having difficulty breathing), bundle him up if it's cold, and get him in the car. He needs to go to the emergency room. Don't forget to figure out what to do with other children, if you have any. Have one parent or caregiver stay at home, call a neighbor to come stay at your home, or get everyone in the car. This may seem obvious, but don't forget about your other kids when one is suddenly ill. This happens! Keep the windows open about one to two inches while you're in the car. Many people who do this arrive at the emergency with a quiet baby with no cough. But don't go home yet! He probably got some blasts of real cold, humid air, is more awake, and has been upright for a period of time, so he may seem fine. The good news is, these babies have a pretty mild degree of croup. But he still needs to be evaluated in the emergency room, and may need to receive some treatments. Doctors may do an X-ray of his neck and chest, to make sure that your baby doesn't have pneumonia, or didn't choke on something earlier that day. Doctors will also measure your baby's oxygen levels, to make sure that he is breathing adequately. There are several treatments that may or may not be given: The first would be a humidification treatment (humidified air with

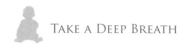

oxygen). This is more intense than the humidification that you would give at home. They may also give a medication called **dexamethasone (Decadron®)**, either as a liquid medicine or a shot. This is a very safe, very commonly used steroid medication, which acts as a very strong, fast-acting anti-inflammatory. It will reduce the swelling in the airway in less than an hour. If your baby seems significantly better after this, he may be sent home. Sometimes you will receive a prescription for liquid steroids to give your baby over the following few days.

If your baby is still having noisy breathing and difficulty after humidifcation and steroids, the doctors may administer a breathing treatment with a medication called **epinephrine**. This will be administered through a **nebulizer**, either as a mask or a plastic tube of air held near your baby's face. The epinephrine (also known as **adrenaline**) is a very strong medication that acts to shrink blood vessels, which leads to reduction in swelling. It acts within a few minutes. Some of the major common side effects of epinephrine are rapid heart rate and rise in blood pressure. Babies can also develop something called a rebound response, whereby the airway will swell several hours after administration of the nebulized epinephrine. This is a reason why many facilities will admit a baby to the hospital after administration of an epinephrine treatment, in order to monitor, and, if necessary, treat a rebound response to the medication.

My baby was born prematurely, and had a breathing tube in his windpipe for three weeks before he went home. Is he more susceptible to develop croup?

Babies who had breathing tubes in their windpipes are not necessarily more susceptible to developing the virus that causes croup *per se*, but they do have a more sensitive airway. The presence of a breathing tube for any length of time in an infant may lead to development of either a scar tissue or minor swelling in the airway. These babies may develop croup-like symptoms (barky cough, noisy breathing) with a cold, as the mucus or swelling present during a cold may irritate the already mildly inflamed and delicate airway. If your baby had a breathing tube placed at any time, for any length of time, she is more susceptible to develop croupy coughs. Treatment in these instances is similar to treatment for croup in general, perhaps with higher vigilance for croup-like symptoms during mild colds.

My baby had croup for the last two nights. He's doing much better, and the barky cough is gone. But now he has a wet, juicy cough. Is this normal?

Think of the swelling that your baby has from croup as a sponge filled with water. As the croup heals (croup cough usually lasts two to three days), the 'water' gets squeezed out. As this happens, the airway swelling goes down, but the tiny mucus glands in the windpipe begin to drain some fluid and mucus. Babies who are recovering from croup often develop a 'wet' cough. They lose the barky/brassy quality, and it begins to sound more like a cough from a cold. This usually lasts for up to a week. Treatment is usually just rest (your child's daycare or preschool will probably not appreciate having your child there, even though he is not really contagious at this point). Another reason to keep your child at home is that, during this healing process, it is possible for this self-limited viral infection to turn into a bacterial infection (requiring antibiotics), or it may progress to bronchitis or pneumonia. If the wet cough persists for more than a week, or if your baby develops a fever, has a change in appetite, or seems lethargic, call your doctor.

My 12-month-old has had croup twice. What can I do to prevent it from happening, and what can I do to prepare for future episodes?

Unfortunately, if your baby has had several episodes of croup, it is highly possible that these will continue. Most children grow out of these by the age of three years, but some children continue to have croup into late childhood. The good news is, your ears will now be trained, and you will likely be able to predict a 'croup night' before it happens. For instance, your child may have a minor cold, but you may hear the faintest of barks before bedtime, or even a slight raspiness in his voice before putting him to bed. In this case, I believe that a preemptive strike is warranted. Get the humidifier on, or even leave your baby's window open a few inches. Some pediatricians are comfortable giving you extra refills of liquid steroids, and may be comfortable letting you give your baby a dose at the earliest sign of croup. In most instances, these two measures can block (or lessen) a croup episode. The croup may still occur, but you may avoid a severe episode, and save you and your child a trip to the emergency room. If you have a baby with a history of multiple episodes of croup, it's a good idea to pack a supply of liquid steroids on long trips away from home.

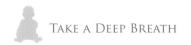

My daughter's worst croup episode was at the age of four years, while we were on a family trip to the desert. The air in the hotel and outside had less than 10% humidity, and it was 2 am on Easter Sunday. We are fortunate enough to be not only experienced with croup, but also both be doctors. My wonderful, loving, sleepless husband was able to find an open pharmacy that night in the middle of the desert. He bought a humidifier and more importantly, did what every doctor shouldn't do: called in a prescription for our own child (for steroids). Two hours later, our child was back to sleep and comfortable. She woke up the next morning completely fine, but we will never travel without steroids again. That said, I don't recommend diagnosing and treating your own child, especially when travelling, but giving one dose of steroids can significantly improve your croupy child's breathing while waiting to get medical attention. Before travelling with a child who's had croup in the past, ask your pediatrician what measures and medications you should take with your child if she develops croup while on the road.

Croup sounds horrible. Is there a vaccine against croup?

Classic croup is caused by several types of viruses, including the cold virus, and **respiratory syncitial virus (RSV)**. The latter virus does have a vaccine, but its administration is limited to high-risk babies (See Section One). While there is no vaccine for the classic viruses that cause croup (most are related to the cold virus), croup can be a complication of the flu virus (for which there is a vaccine every year, recommended annually for all infants over six months). The majority of babies with croup are treated at home, and most kids bounce back to good health within a few days. Most do not need to go to the emergency room (especially if you've had a baby with one episode of croup), and very rarely do they need to be admitted to a hospital.

There is, however a vaccine for an illess which is much more serious and life-threatening, called **epiglottitis**. This is a bacterial infection caused by *haemophilus influenzae*. When the epiglottis becomes infected with this organism, it swells very rapidly, leading to sudden breathing trouble, drooling, hoarseness, and respiratory distress. Children try to breathe by sitting up, and leaning their neck and chin forward (the 'sniffing' position). Let them stay this way if it makes them more comfortable. They may have a cough as well, but it will sound weaker than the loud, barky cough of croup. Epiglottitis has been nearly completely eradicated, due to widespread immunization with the H. influenzae type "B" (HiB) vaccine, the first dose of which is given at the age of two months. This was a life-threatening illness, which, thanks to vaccination, has become nearly non-existent.

What other vaccinations does my baby need before her first birthday?

While many vaccines may seem unnecessary, and some may have risks, vaccines are necessary. They are not only necessary for your baby's health and safety, but they are also necessary for public health safety. "**Herd immunity**" (yes, we are still animals, in herds, after all), is the concept that if all are immunized in a given community, a particular disease will be eradicated. Conversely, lack of immunization of *some* members of the 'herd' will lead to resurgence of a given disease. This happens because people who are not immunized may spread disease to others who are either (1) not yet fully immunized, (2) not immunized at all or (3) have weakened immune systems (such as infants, elderly, or those with chronic illness). We have seen this with pertussis (the 'P' in DTaP, causing whooping cough), measles (the 'M' in MMR) and mumps (the other 'M' in MMR). There have also been reported cases of *hemophilus influenzae* meningitis, leading to irreversible nervous system problems such as developmental delays, and permanent deafness. These diseases, which in the recent past were those of developing nations or underserved communities, have become ailments of the wealthy. But these diseases are just as aggressive to all comers, and do not act more kindly to those with deep pockets. Some of the most affluent, educated communities in the United States have experienced large outbreaks of preventable diseases. Vaccines used to carry some risks due to mercury content, and mercury's negative effect on the developing nervous system. This theory was disproven, and nonetheless, there is no mercury in vaccines being administered today. Concerns that vaccine use is a cause for the increased incidence of autism continues to be an area of heated debate, but most evidence for this has been disproven.

According to the CDC guidelines, the vaccine schedule between ages three and 12 months is as follows:

Four months:

❖ DTaP (second dose) (Diphtheria/Tetanus/Pertussis)
❖ Hib (second dose)(Hemophilus influenzae b)

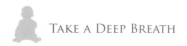
❖ Pneumococcal vaccine (second dose)

❖ IPV (second dose) (Inactivated poliovirus)

Six months:

❖ DTaP (third dose)

❖ Hib (third dose)

❖ Pneumococcal vaccine (third dose)

❖ IPV (third dose) (may be given between six and 18 months)

❖ Hepatitis B (second dose) (may be given between six and 18 months)

❖ Influenza (yearly after first dose) (baby's first influenza vaccine is given as two separate vaccines, each administered 30 days apart)

12 months:

❖ Hib (fourth dose)(may be given between 12 and 15 months)

❖ Pneumococcal vaccine (fourth dose) (may be given between 12 and 15 months)

❖ MMR (Measles, mumps, rubella) (first dose) (may be given between 12 and 15 months)

❖ Varicella (may be given between 12 and 15 months)

❖ Hepatitis A (two doses between 12 and 23 months, at least six months apart)

THE BIG PICTURE

Croup is a commonly encountered viral illness of the respiratory system, and can be present in the early months of life. The cough of croup has a classic sound, and once your baby has had an episode (and the diagnosis was confirmed by your doctor), you may expect it to happen again. While you can be prepared for future episodes, I still recommend that you call your doctor (or bring your child to an emergency room) to confirm that it is indeed croup. There are very rare disorders that can mimic croup, and these need to be addressed by a specialist. In medicine, there is a saying, 'When you hear hoof beats, think horses, not zebras'. In other words, 'common things happen commonly'. However, rare things ('zebras') do happen, so medical attention is still warranted, even for the most routine croup episode. You may not need to bring your baby to the doctor's office, but a phone call is important.

Most babies who are recovering from croup develop a wet, mucousy cough. This may linger for several days, but if your baby seems ill, with fever, lethargy, breathing trouble, or loss of appetite, call your doctor right away.

Severe croup is rare, and it does require more urgent, aggressive medical attention. If your baby has a barky cough and seems to have trouble breathing, or if he has a blue discoloration on his lips or skin, bring him to the emergency room or call 911. If, while you are driving to the emergency room, your baby seems dramatically better, don't turn around and go home. He was sick enough to go there, and he deserves a thorough evaluation.

Stay up to date with your child's immunization schedule. There are many life-threatening, preventable illnesses that vaccines work against. Staying on schedule with these will protect your baby and those around her. On the other hand, if you have 'opted out' of vaccinating your child, but change your mind to do so, it is never too late! Your doctor can get your child back on a schedule, and he can still become fully immunized.

DON'T WORRY

If your baby has a mild cold, with a clear runny nose, mild stuffiness, and no or minimal fever, but wakes in the night barking like a seal, take a good look at her. Is she struggling to breathe, or just coughing loudly? If it's just the loud, harsh cough, it is likely croup. Stay calm! Your baby will surely sense your anxiety, which may make her breathing more labored. Bring her outside, or to a humid area. If her croup is mild, her symptoms should subside in five to ten minutes. She may still have the cough, but it will be less 'harsh' in nature. Your baby may become more relaxed and less agitated. Get the humidifier for her room. Give your doctor a call to see if you need to come in to the office or emergency room. Most babies with croup will be dramatically better in the morning (after they've slept, but you've been awake, of course). It is still a good idea to let your doctor know, even if she seems fine in the morning. You may be able to prevent another night similar to it.

If your baby wakes suddenly at night (or any time of day, for that matter) with a loud, brassy cough, and has any sign of trouble breathing or blue discoloration to the skin, go to the nearest emergency room or call 911. If your baby has not been vaccinated with the HiB vaccine, and develops a sudden episode of breathing trouble, drooling, and cough, call 911. It may be epiglottitis. Let him stay in the position that is most comfortable for him until help arrives.

TO-DO LIST: RESPIRATORY ILLNESSES IN BABIES: CROUP AND CRUD

1. If you hear your baby coughing suddenly in the middle of the night, and you think he may have a new pet seal in his bed, it may be croup.

2. If it's just a cough, with no breathing difficulty, try humidity — either outside, in a steamed bathroom, or with a room humidifier.

3. If your baby has breathing difficulty with a cough, call 911 or bring her to the emergency room. While you are driving to the emergency room, keep the car windows open about one to two inches.

4. Don't forget about the other children in the house. It may seem obvious when reading this, but it's surprisingly easy to do this in an emergency.

5. It's always good to have a back-up plan in event of any child's emergency, whether it's a breathing problem or a broken limb. Neighbor? Other parent or caregiver? This designated person needs to be available at any time, and must be willing and able to take care of your other children in a flash, especially in the middle of the night (when the majority of emergencies occur). This person should be designated *before* an emergency occurs.

6. If your baby has had two or more episodes of croup, check with your pediatrician about having a refill of oral medication (steroids) at home, to be used until medical care is given.

7. Check with your doctor about safety, administration, side effects, and risks of steroids. Many people worry about side effects such as growth delay and hormonal imbalance with steroid use. While there are known (and legitimate) risks and side

effects, short-term use of steroids has very few long-term risks. Common short-term risks include jitteriness, stomach irritation, blood sugar elevation, and increase in appetite.

8. Steroid dosing needs to be precise, and may need to be tapered (stopped gradually). Very short-term use usually does not require tapering, but always check with your doctor about exact dosing and possible need for gradually reducing the dose. Stopping steroids suddenly may lead to dangerous rebound reactions, especially if given for several days at high doses.

9. Keep your baby on schedule for his immunizations. Make sure that older children and adults who have direct contact with your baby are also immunized.

Source for Respiratory Illnesses in Babies:

www.mayoclinic.com/health/croup/DS00312

Chapter Thirteen
Nebulizers: What's in Them?

Some babies who develop respiratory infections will have prolonged coughing or wheezing, weeks after the illness has cleared. He may seem fine all day, but may be up all night coughing, long after a cold or a cough has subsided. You may bring him to the doctor for a check-up, and your doctor may hear wheezing. Does this mean your baby has asthma? Not necessarily. More likely, your baby has something called **Reactive Airway Disease (RAD)**. It is not really a 'disease' in the true sense of the word, but it is an entity whereby a cold turns into prolonged periods of coughing and wheezing, long after the cold itself subsides. RAD is just that, a 'reactive' airway. The airway 'reacts' to any inflammatory process, which is most often a cold or a cough. The 'reaction' that forms is inflammation (swelling) of the windpipe and/or lower air passages such as the **bronchi** (small air passages between the windpipe and lungs) or the lungs themselves. Many babies who have RAD eventually grow out of it by the end of preschool, but some go on to develop true **asthma** (a chronic inflammatory disease of the bronchi and lungs). There is also an increased likelihood for babies with RAD to eventually have evidence of environmental allergies. Doctors often give babies with RAD prescriptions for nebulizers, either to be used on a regular basis, or to be used during or after respiratory illnesses. If your baby needs to receive nebulizer therapy, it's good to know what you are giving your baby, why you are giving it, and how to use it safely and effectively.

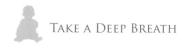

My nine-month-old had a bad cold three weeks ago, and she continues to cough all night. She's no longer sick, her doctor says it's not bronchitis or pneumonia, but he recommended nebulized breathing treatments. What are these?

Babies and young toddlers are not capable of receiving inhalers (the hand-held 'puffers' used by asthmatic children or adults). Inhaled medications need to be administered via a **nebulizer**. In hospitals, nebulizers may be attached from breathing machines or oxygen supply systems attached to the walls or anesthesia carts. But home nebulizers (or nebulizers in doctors' offices) are portable, and consist of a small motor, a battery or electrical source, and a compressed air chamber. Tubing is attached to the machine, and this tubing is attached to a small hose-like apparatus or infant-sized plastic mask. The medication (in liquid form) is placed in a small chamber between the machine and the mask. The forced air passes from the machine through the plastic tubing, and enables the liquid medication to become aerosolized, and thus inhaled in a cool-steam form.

Are you serious? My baby won't even let me brush her two teeth! You think she'll sit still for a breathing treatment?

Indeed, nobody said it would be easy. But this is one of those 'who's the boss?' times. You know your baby best, so you will have to be creative in what will work for your sanity and efficacy in giving these treatments. These are not true inhalers, so you don't have to worry about timing your baby's breathing, or getting the tubing or mask directly into his mouth. This is an inhaled steam-form of a medication. The mask and tubing need to be in the vicinity of her nose and mouth — the closer the better, of course, but start by getting her accustomed to the treatments. And crying counts as breathing. Even if you do a 'blow-by' treatment, where the mask is at least near your baby's face, some of the steam is breathed in, and this is a good start. There is no best technique, but here are some options:

❖ Let your baby hold the tubing or mask herself, before turning on the machine. She can even put it near or in her mouth. It wont hurt anything.

❖ Show your baby how you breathe the mask or bring the tubing to your mouth. Let her try first, before the machine or steam comes out.

❖ Let the steam blow around the room first. Put your hand through it, to show her that it doesn't hurt. Let her 'touch' the steam first.

❖ Have your baby sit in her high chair. This is a familiar place, and hopefully has positive associations. Put some toys on the tray. Distract, distract, distract.

❖ Have your baby sit on your lap in a quiet, comfortable room. Unfortunately, many of the portable nebulizer machines are quite noisy, but minimizing ambient noise (or siblings) may help.

❖ Make a breathing song for your baby, or play a favorite CD or read a book.

❖ Television/handheld technology of choice. This is where you may want to put the 'No TV under age 2 years' plan out the window. You've got to get ready for work, get your child ready for daycare, and complete a 15-minute breathing treatment before 8 am. Practicality wins on this one.

My doctor prescribed steroid nebulizer treatments for my baby. She said I should give them three times per day when she has a cold, and for a few weeks afterwards. Does this sound right?

Steroid nebulizers are commonly given to babies and toddlers with reactive airway disease. The medical term for the drug most commonly used is **budesonide**, and the trade name is **Pulmicort®**. Inhaled steroids do not work acutely, which means that they will not improve symptoms of coughing or wheezing after one treatment. It can take from one day to two weeks before the anti-inflammatory effect of inhaled steroids begins to work. Budesonide for infants and children is prepared in individual plastic packs of liquid medication, which is then poured into the nebulizer container. It comes in various dosage levels. When the nebulizer machine is turned on, the compressed air will turn this liquid into steam, and the steroid can be inhaled. Many babies with reactive airway disease will stay on 'maintenance' steroid nebulizer therapy through the respiratory infection season, depending on how severe their reactive airway disease symptoms are. This daily treatment may prevent exacerbation of chronic coughing and wheezing. Some doctors will recommend maintenance as a low-dose (once per day) steroid inhalation, with increase in frequency (up to four times per day) during and shortly after acute respiratory illnesses. Always check with your doctor before you increase or decrease the frequency of steroid inhalers.

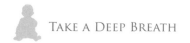
Many parents are concerned about the safety of steroid inhalers, and the degree that the steroids are absorbed into the bloodstream. This is a very reasonable concern. Studies have shown that there is some absorption into the bloodstream with steroid inhalers. Go over details of techniques for minimizing side effects of steroid inhalation with your doctor, and don't hesitate to ask questions. Most children will not have any sudden side effects from these inhalers (except for maybe being angry at you for making them do a breathing treatment), but there are some potential concerns, such as steroid exposure to the eyes, risks of fungal infections in the mouth, and potential for growth delays. But before nixing the idea of inhaled steroids, talk to your doctor about your concerns. The risks and side effects are primarily dependent on dosing, frequency, and duration of use. And as with any treatment, you will also have to weigh the risks of a baby who is struggling to breathe, cant stop coughing and is wheezing against the risks of the medications to treat this.

My doctor has also recommended using a medication called albuterol when my baby gets sick. Isn't this for kids with asthma?

Albuterol is a medication commonly used to treat wheezing seen in asthmatics. It acts by opening up the small airways (**bronchi**) during an asthma attack. It also works to keep these bronchi open as a maintenance medication. In children with reactive airway disease (their airways 'react' to colds and coughs by becoming swollen and closed), albuterol acts similarly, by opening up the closed, swollen airways. Infants and children are most commonly prescribed a medication call **levalbuterol** (the common trade name is **Xopenex®**). It can be used once a day as a 'maintenance' inhalation when the child is well, or it can be used up to four times per day when a child is ill. It can be mixed together with an inhaled steroid to be given as one breathing treatment. There are no steroids in this medication, so concerns about steroid absorption is not an issue. But this is a strong drug, with its own side effects. Drugs in this family may cause increase in heart rate, jitteriness, or shaking. In infants and young children, it may make them a

IF YOUR BABY NEEDS NEBULIZER TREATMENTS, IT DOES NOT NECESSARILY MEAN THAT SHE HAS OR WILL HAVE ASTHMA bit hyper and wild. If your child seems extremely agitated (beyond just being upset from the nebulizer itself) after albuterol treatments, let your doctor know right away. You may need to lower the dose, or change the medication. For the most part, this drug, as well as inhaled steroids, is very well tolerated in most infants and children. And unlike inhaled steroids, the beneficial effects of inhaled albuterol are seen almost immediately — reduced cough, more comfortable breathing, and less wheezing, even after one treatment. The biggest battle with albuterol is usually getting used to the nebulizer itself. But, as with most things, once you and your baby get into a breathing treatment routine, it becomes easier.

My doctor recommended that I should combine both budesonide and levalbuterol for nebulizer treatments. Does this make sense?

Yes. These medications work differently, so it is reasonable for your baby to receive both. The budesonide (Pulmicort®) is an inhaled steroid, and works by reducing the inflammation/swelling in the airway. The levalbuterol (Xopenex®) is a **bronchodilator**, which acts to open up ('dilate') the small air passages between the windpipe and lungs (bronchi). Using both does not mean that you are giving a double dose of medication, as they each work differently. They often provide significantly more benefit by working together. Many doctors recommend that your baby stay on Pulmicort® nebulizers throughout the cold season, and that you add Xopenex® during and after colds or coughs.

My baby uses inhaled nebulizer treatments during colds. Last week, she became really sick, and I couldn't get her cough better with the nebulizer treatment. I brought her to the emergency room and they gave her a nebulizer with epinephrine. It worked great, but they said I couldn't get a prescription for this at home. Why not?

Epinephrine (also known as **adrenaline**) is an extremely powerful medication that acts to shrink blood vessels, thereby causing significant reduction in swelling. It works quickly and effectively in liquid form when given via a nebulizer for airway swelling. Patients (from babies to adults) need to be monitored very closely during and after receiving such a medication for several reasons. First of all, it may cause very rapid heart rate or elevation in blood pressure. It can also lead to a 'rebound' response in

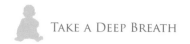

the airway. This means that several hours after receiving this treatment, the airway can swell even more. Many babies who receive epinephrine nebulizers are admitted to the hospital for observation, or are at least observed for several hours to monitor for a relapse of breathing problems. Epinephrine nebulizers need to be given in a hospital setting.

THE BIG PICTURE

Nebulizer treatments are being increasingly used as a treatment for breathing problems in children of all ages, even babies. If your baby has chronic coughing (usually for more than two to three weeks) following respiratory illnesses, or if your baby's colds are associated with severe coughing or wheezing, your doctor may recommend a trial of nebulizer treatments at home. While this may seem daunting, you will soon notice that the benefits (nights without coughing) outweigh the nuisance and concerns surrounding the treatments. If your baby needs nebulizer treatments due to respiratory illnesses, this does not necessarily mean that he will go on to develop asthma (although he is at a slightly higher risk than the general population, it is not directly correlated with lifelong need for breathing treatments). The vast majority of infants and toddlers who need nebulizer treatments eventually grow out of it.

Initial use of nebulizers can be quite frustrating and exhausting. But I'll say it: take a deep breath. Take a break. Some babies really go for it, and some will have no part of it. You may have to be a bit creative on this one. Some companies even make colorful masks with animal faces to keep your baby interested. The steam that comes out has essentially no smell or taste, so it shouldn't be that disconcerting to your little one. The noise of the machine seems to be most bothersome to many of the young children. You can try covering it with a blanket to mute it out a little, or play some loud music for distraction. When all else fails: TV, favorite DVD, or handheld technological device of choice may be used.

The medications in the nebulizer treatments are shown to be safe in infants and children. Potential side effects need to be reviewed with your doctor, and don't hesitate to ask questions if concerns come up. Many babies with reactive airway disease (RAD) in infancy 'grow out' of it as they get older. While some go on to develop true 'asthma', the majority will grow out of RAD, as well as their need for nebulizers, before kindergarten.

DON'T WORRY

If your baby seems to have colds that never end, or colds that turn into relentless coughing long after the colds are done, she may have an entity called reactive airway disease (RAD). It is surprisingly common, especially as babies reach their first birthday. Do not panic. It does not necessarily mean that your baby is asthmatic, chronically ill, or prone to pneumonia. It does, however mean that you need to be vigilant when she does get cold, that you need to keep track of her medication schedule, and that other caregivers need to learn how to administer nebulizer treatments. Don't get too frustrated if your baby rejects the nebulizer to begin with. Keep trying. Distraction is a big help.

WORRY

If your baby is having severe wheezing, coughing to the point of difficulty breathing or vomiting, or if your baby is having breathing trouble, using her chest or stomach muscles to breathe, or has any blue discoloration, call 911 or bring her to the emergency room. If she has been using nebulizers for chronic coughing or wheezing, she may need to be treated with a stronger nebulizer treatment, such as epinephrine. This cannot be done at home.

TO-DO LIST: NEBULIZERS: WHAT'S IN THEM?

1. If your baby has a chronic cough (greater than two weeks) following a cold, let your doctor know. He may have some degree of reactive airway disease (RAD), which can be treated with nebulizers.

2. If your baby does require nebulizers during or after colds, it may not necessarily mean that she will go on to develop asthma.

3. If your baby does receive a prescription to use nebulizers, ask questions. It is important for you to know what you are giving your baby, how the medications will help your baby, and how best to administer the medication for best results.

4. Administering nebulizer treatments to infants takes some practice. If your doctor's office has a nebulizer, ask them to demonstrate how to use it.

5. Give it some time at home. Do not expect great results on the first few tries. You may have to try several techniques to see which one your baby takes to.

6. The medicines for nebulizers come in prescription form, and can be bought at standard pharmacies. The machines, however, are either rented or bought at medical supply companies. Your doctor should be able to guide you to the right sources for these.

7. The most commonly used nebulizer for babies with coughing and wheezing is albuterol (or levalbuterol, which is very similar). This medication works by opening up the small air passages between the windpipe and the lungs.

8. A second commonly used medication is budesonide (Pulmicort®), which is an inhaled steroid.

9. Many doctors will recommend using budesonide on a regular basis, especially during cold season, and then adding albuterol when your child is sick.

10. Ask your doctor about the side effects of nebulizer medications.

11. If your baby does not seem to be getting better from nebulizer treatments, call your doctor or bring him to the emergency room.

12. The strongest nebulizer medication, epinephrine, can only be used in a hospital or emergency room. This medication works very quickly and effectively, but your child needs to be under direct medical supervision when receiving this.

Sources for Nebulizers:
www.kidshealth.org/parent/medical/asthma/inhaler_nebulizer
www.ncbi.nlm.nih.gov/pubmedhealth/pmh0000234 (levalbuterol)
www.ncbi.nlm.nih.gov/pubmedhealth/pmh0001064 (budesonide)
www.drugs.com/cdi/epinephrine-nebulizer-solution

Chapter Fourteen
Clear the Air for the First Year

Babies under one year are still very sensitive to environmental irritants, and their increased mobility puts them more at risk for exposure to toxins, both in and out of the home. While their immune system and respiratory system are more mature than those of a young infant, they are still vulnerable to illness and inflammation from exposure to multiple pollutants. After the first few months of life, most parents are eager to bring their baby out and about, perhaps take a plane trip, vacation, visit friends, go to parks, or join playgroups. This is a wonderful time for babies to begin more social interactions, both with adults as well as with other children. What are some of the effects the environment (both indoor and outdoor) can have on your baby's breathing? Does global warming have an impact? Or living in a big city? What about living close to a freeway?

I worry about all the scares we hear about our horrible environment and all the toxins to which our kids are exposed. Is air quality much worse than it was when we were kids?

While there are more and more toxins that we are now finding to be linked to hormonal abnormalities and cancer, you will be pleasantly surprised to know that the air quality in the United States is significantly better than it was ten, twenty, and even thirty years ago. We can thank the Environmental Protection Agency (EPA) for this. Back in the 1940's and 1950's, air pollution was at an all-time high in the U.S., and people were developing chronic lung disease, and even dying from the polluted air, particularly in industrial areas. The public health concerns of air pollution alerted federal agencies, and in 1963 the Clean Air Act was passed. This

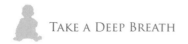

was the first step in providing funding to study ways to clean up the air. In 1970, Congress passed stronger regulations regarding air pollution, giving the EPA the responsibility for multiple programs related to the Clean Air Act. In 1990, there were even more regulations passed regarding the EPA's authority to implement and enforce major regulations regarding tangible approaches to reduce air pollution. This authority enabled the EPA to set limits on certain air pollutants from sources such as chemical plants, utilities, and steel mills, to ensure basic health and environmental protection for all Americans. The EPA still continues to make efforts to improve air quality. In 2010, it provided grants to help projects that reduce harmful diesel emissions from vehicles like school buses, garbage trucks, construction equipment, marine vessels, and trains. It also proposed a mandatory reporting system for greenhouse gas emissions, which include carbon dioxide, methane, nitrous oxide, hydrofluorocarbons, perfluorocarbons, and sulfur hexafluoride, from large companies. They have also instituted a program where schools located in urban areas or near industrial facilities undergo outdoor monitoring of toxic air pollutants for 60-day periods, in an effort to establish a more regulated reduction of specific pollutants to which children are exposed.

So is air pollution really down? Has this been shown? There is so much in the news about global warming and toxins, it's hard to believe that any improvements have been made.
Here's the good news: There has been a quantifiable reduction in major air pollutants in the U.S. since 1997 (seven years after the revised Clean Air Act went into effect). The EPA keeps close records of average annual pollutant levels across the country, and the four 'major' air pollutants (carbon monoxide, sulfur dioxide, nitrous dioxide, and particulate matter), have decreased nationwide since the late 1990's.

Is air pollution really linked to respiratory illnesses?
Yes. Many large, population-based studies in the United States have confirmed association between air pollution and asthma, bronchitis, respiratory illnesses, and even ear infections. With the reduction in air pollution, there has been a reduction in respiratory illnesses. This has been shown in other countries, as well. After the fall of the Berlin Wall in 1989, more stringent rules on emissions from chemical

plants in East Germany were instituted. Several years later, large East German populations in these industrialized towns showed significant reduction in degree and frequency of respiratory illnesses and infections, mostly due to improved air quality.

It's great to hear that the nation's air quality has improved, but I live in a big city. It certainly does not seem to have clean air. Is there anything I can do to protect my baby?

While it's nice to hear that statistics are better overall, it may not be the case in your city or town, and the optimistic numbers may do nothing for your particular situation. There are no miracle answers for this, short of moving to a rural area or wearing a gas mask. In this situation, all you can do is your part in keeping the air clean. This may sound trite, but if you don't own or regulate chemical plants, construction sites, or car companies, all you can do is what you think is right for you, your family, and your community. Whether it's driving a hybrid or electric vehicle, carpooling, driving less, or mowing your lawn less often, there are ways each individual can contribute to cleaner air quality.

I live in an apartment and my neighbor smokes. Can this affect my baby?

Yes. Especially if air vents or heating systems are centralized in buildings, fumes from other apartments can track through to other units. Toxins can even penetrate through walls and ceilings over time. Some towns and cities have tried to issue ordinances about smoking bans in apartment complexes, however these regulations are certainly few and far between. Direct effects from cigarette smoke from *a neighbor* are difficult to document. While it is well known that infants exposed to cigarette smoke are more at risk to develop chronic respiratory conditions, it is hard to prove that exposure from a neighbor can cause such direct impact. While it is likely that there are some negative effects from indirect exposure, those effects are hard to measure, and even harder to regulate. A recent study in the most respected pediatrics journal showed that children who live in apartment complexes had much higher levels of measurable toxins from second hand smoke than those living in single-family homes, even if nobody in their own apartment was a smoker. Possible sources are seepage through the walls or ventilation systems.

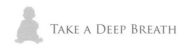

There is a great park in my town, but it's close to a major highway.
Should I avoid bringing my baby there?

While studies have shown that children who live close to major roadways are at
increased risk for developing chronic respiratory illnesses such as asthma, none have
shown that occasional proximity has long term downsides. If you live in an urban
area, or an area that has many major roads, your air quality is likely to be worse than
it would be if you lived in a remote location. But the difference between being five
miles away from a roadway and a mile away from a roadway, certainly for an afternoon, has a miniscule difference in air quality. In other words, if you live anywhere
near that great park, your air quality is probably not much better than the air quality at the park itself. Let your baby enjoy the afternoon at the park.

Global warming terrifies me. Is my baby going to be sicker because of it?

While books, movies, and careers are spent investigating the impact that global
warming may or may not have on our health as well as on the planet, the data are
variable regarding the impact that global warming may or may not have on respiratory illnesses. Some studies have shown that average increase in annual temperature
has no impact on respiratory illnesses (including ear infections, which may be considered a respiratory illness, as they often originate from colds and nasal congestion).
Some studies have shown that rise in temperature, increased humidity, and tropical
rains are linked to increase in multiple infectious diseases, including respiratory
illnesses. While pollutants in and of themselves have been shown to be associated
with respiratory illnesses, the jury is out regarding the direct connection between
respiratory illness and average annual temperature.

We are planning a six-hour flight with our five-month-old. It happens to be
over a major holiday, during the cold and flu season. What can we do to
minimize her chances of getting sick?

Unfortunately, winter holiday travel with an infant is a bit like a game of Roulette,
or Poker, or Slots. Babies can get up to ten colds per year, most of which also occur
in the winter. Adults also get a few colds per year, most of which occur also in the
winter, and are well timed during the holiday season. So you don't need to be a
statistics whiz to figure out that there is a decent chance that your baby may have

a cold the week you plan to fly. That said, the BEST way to minimize your baby's chances of getting sick during travel is for her to be well before travel. This is no easy task. But this may be a time where you may want to decide not to bring your brand new bundle of joy to the office holiday party, where she will be passed around like a fruit cake, kissed by strangers (or at least strange co-workers), and unduly exposed to everyone's lingering or imminent cold virus. And remember, many of your co-workers either haven't gotten around to, or have chosen not to, receive a flu vaccine. Your baby is too young to be immunized, so she is at a high risk to be exposed to and develop the flu virus in this setting. It's also good, in general, the week or two before a flight, to keep your baby as routinized as possible, and keep her hydrated. It is also critical that you and your family stay healthy even if you are stressed, whether it's from life with your new baby, work, family, holiday shopping, weather change, or all of the above. If you get run down or sick, your baby will most likely also become unwell. Take extra good care of yourself (and spouse) during this time.

Assuming that the stars have aligned, and you, your family, and your baby are healthy, now you need to stay that way while you and 250 of your closest friends breathe in that lovely recycled dry air at 35,000 feet. Here are some tips for baby's health in the air:

1. Buy your baby her own ticket. Not only is this the safest way to travel (your baby doesn't sit in your lap in a car, why should she on an airplane), it is also the healthiest. She will have her own space (her infant car seat), minimizing her ability to touch all of the seats and armrests around her, she will be able to sleep more comfortably, and you can still take her out from time to time. She will also be more concealed from her neighbor's seat. The Federal Aviation Association (FAA) requires that infants in car seats should be given window seats. Since you will be sitting next to her (and stuck with a middle seat for this and all foreseeable future flights), there is no chance that one of those sneezing passengers will be next to her.

2. Bring extra baby wipes. Hand sanitizers are not considered safe for infants. Hand sanitizers contain high levels of alcohol (ethanol). Babies can lick their hands after you clean them, and ingest small, although measurable, amounts of alcohol.

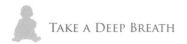

3. Bring saline nasal spray (don't share these with family members — you should each have your own bottle, labeled with each person's name). Spray your baby's nose once or twice before take-off, and every two hours (when she's awake) during the flight. *Now* aren't you glad she's restrained in her car seat?

4. Spray your own nose as well, every two hours. Feel free to use the airplane lavatory to do this in private.

5. Extra hydration, not only for your baby, but also for you, especially if you are breastfeeding.

6. Do not drink alcohol, especially if you are breastfeeding.

7. If your baby is a bit congested before the flight, ask your doctor if it's safe to bring **oxymetazoline (Afrin®)**. This is a nasal decongestant spray. It will help to prevent the congestion from turning into a sinus infection or a worsening cold. If you use it, give your baby one or two sprays (or you can turn the bottle upside down to create a dropper effect) right before takeoff. You need to do this only once, as its effect lasts for 12 hours. It's a good idea to give a few sprays of saline before giving Afrin®, in order to flush out any of the mucus that's sitting inside your baby's nose. If your baby is stuffy after the flight, you may continue using Afrin®, but a maximum of two sprays, two times per day, for two days (2-2-2).

8. Don't forget to place all spray bottles in easily accessible clear plastic bags in your carry-on bag. These will need to pass through security separate from the rest of your carry-on items. As of 2011, three-ounce liquid bottles and medicines are approved for carry-on travel.

9. Bring infant **acetominophen** (and **ibuprofen** for babies six months and over) in your bag of liquid carry-ons.

10. Wash your hands often or use baby wipes or hand sanitizer. It isn't just your baby and strangers who carry germs.

THE BIG PICTURE

Infants in the first year of life are still susceptible to respiratory irritants such as air pollution, cigarette smoke, and other people's viruses. They have slightly better ability than their newborn counterparts to handle these exposures, however, they are still tiny, vulnerable creatures. The good news is that the air is actually cleaner than it was when we were kids. It may not seem so, especially when there seems to be daily discoveries regarding newly found toxins in foods, toys, and even sippy cups. But when we are talking specifically about air quality (meaning amounts of toxic air pollutants), the numbers are favorable, throughout the whole United States and many parts of the world. In many ways, indoor pollutants or contaminants, such as fumes from old lead paint, dust in the ventilation system, or second-hand smoke, are more concerning than outdoor pollutants for infants, older children, and adults alike. Protecting your baby from any undesirable exposure is what every parent wants, but the reality is that the world in which we live is imperfect. Minimize exposure to any kind of smoke, and also to other sick people, especially in enclosed settings. Saline nasal spray is still the best way to 'flush out' any potentially irritating substances. Think of it as a bath or shower for the respiratory system. If your baby is exposed to sick people, flush out her nose with saline when you get home. Her nose probably contains some viral or bacterial particles from exposure to someone's sneeze or cough, and flushing out the nose can minimize her chances of becoming sick. It is also great to do the same during travel, especially on long airplane flights.

DON'T WORRY

If you live in a big city, or near a major roadway, it is likely that the air that you and your baby breathe is not as clean as it would be if you lived in a rural area, away from major industry. But, overall, air quality (measured as levels of major pollutants annually) has improved significantly over the last 15 years, and continues to do so each year. If you are concerned, this is a good time to see what you and your family can do to minimize your contribution to pollution — reduce car travel when possible, rake the leaves instead of having someone use a leaf blower (they are notorious for emitting noxious fumes into the environment), consider alternative energy sources, and most definitely do not smoke.

WORRY

Most concerning environmental exposures occur indoors, and are usually due to exposure to sick people. If your baby is under six months and has not received the flu vaccine, she is especially vulnerable to developing the flu if exposed to sick adults (who may not have received the vaccine either). Keep exposure to large groups to a minimum, especially during winter months. This is not to say I recommend avoiding family get-togethers, but perhaps pass on the office party the week before a trip to that family gathering — it may increase the chances of you and your family actually making it there in good health.

TO-DO LIST: CLEAR THE AIR FOR THE FIRST YEAR

1. Do not quarantine your baby. Enjoy some fresh air! (It really is fresher than you think.)

2. Most 'toxic' air exposure for babies will occur indoors, and from individuals with respiratory illnesses.

3. If your baby has not yet had a flu vaccine, minimize close crowd exposure during flu season.

4. Prepare, prepare, prepare for airplane travel. Bring hydration items such as nasal saline and water, pain medication, along with baby wipes on the flight.

5. If at all possible, purchase a seat on the plane for your baby. It is not only safer, but it is also healthier.

6. Do your part to minimize air pollution.

Sources for Clearing the Air for the First Year:
www.epa.gov/air/caa/peg/understand
www.pediatrics.org/cgi/doi/10.1542/peds.2010-2046

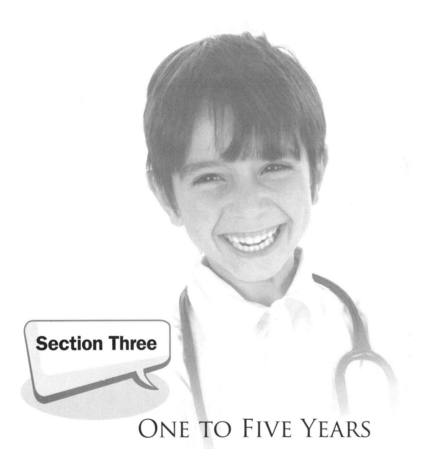

ONE TO FIVE YEARS

The toddler and preschool years are exciting ones. Your completely dependent infant seems to morph before your eyes into an independent being. Developmental changes are enormous in these years, as your baby becomes a child.

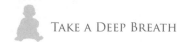

He evolves from crawling on all fours to a boy standing tall. She progresses from a cherubic angel in a stroller to a princess with magic powers. From a breathing standpoint, there are also many changes. Upright creatures can better tolerate breathing difficulties than those who cannot hold their head up, sit, or stand. But as your baby becomes a child, she will encounter new breathing issues, some of which are progressions from infancy, and some of which are unique to toddlers. A large portion of these breathing issues will be related to exposure at playgroups, daycare, or preschool. Some issues will be related to changes in her anatomy, and some will be related to changes in her immune system. In these chapters, I will walk you through the toddler years, giving explanations for new breathing concerns, and recommendations for treatment, and, more importantly, prevention.

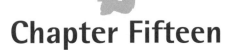

Chapter Fifteen

Stuffy Nose/Runny Nose/ Sinusitis — From Friends and Foes

Around the age of three years, virtually all children join some kind of daycare, playgroup, or preschool. Or they may have a sibling or two. Many of these children are with someone other than their parent for most of the day, possibly in large groups of other children with one or two adult caregivers, be they daycare providers, babysitters, or teachers. Children are explorers at this age (this may explain why Dora the Explorer is so popular with tots), and they love to touch everything — with their hands, their feet, their noses, and mouths. Nothing is gross to a two-year-old. They live for 'gross'. With the thrill of saliva-coated fingers in a friend's mouth can lead to more colds, chronic runny noses, and even sinusitis. While colds and runny noses are common, and usually run their course on their own, sinusitis is a potentially serious problem that may warrant medical attention. This chapter will give some tips on how to keep even the most adventurous toddler's colds to a minimum, what 'chronic' really means for a chronic runny nose, and what sinusitis is, how it is diagnosed by your doctor, how it is treated, and what you can do to clear it fast and prevent it from coming back.

My 18-month-old seems to have a runny nose all fall and winter.
Is he sick? Is there anything I can do to get rid of this?
Many toddlers, especially during the first half of the school year, seem to have chronic runny noses. There may be some days when it seems a little better, but there are

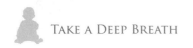
more days than not when it's running. Many parents will report that this starts sometime around the first week of October, and can last through the winter and early spring. The reason for the October start is that the cold viruses from the start of school need to simmer and spread for the first two to three weeks, so it is very typical for runny noses to start a few weeks after Labor Day, coinciding with the start of school. And they tend to perpetuate, as they are passed around from one classroom to the next. For the most part, little treatment or concern is warranted. Assuming your child is not coughing, having green or yellow drainage, acting irritable, or running a fever, he can go about his daily routine. Many will be concerned about whether or not the runny nose is contagious. This is very hard to determine, but a good rule of thumb is that the first few days of any new symptom (runny nose, cough, or sneezing) tend to be highly contagious.

To treat the runny nose, good old nasal saline at the beginning of the day, in the middle of the day if your child is home, and before bedtime will flush out the clear mucus, and minimize the chances of it becoming thicker and more bothersome. No cold medication or antibiotics are necessary. Keep your child's hands clean as much as possible. Hand washing (with soap) is one of the best ways to cut down on colds, any time of year. And keep those clean hands out of her nose, and the noses of her friends. If you are on the go, hand sanitizer or infant wipes are a close second to soap and a sink.

My two-year-old's nose runs all day (and so does she), but at night she's very stuffy and uncomfortable. It's interfering with her sleep. Is there a medication I can give her?

If a runny nose leads to nasal stuffiness and congestion at night, consider using a cool mist humidifier in your child's bedroom. This will help prevent the mucus from becoming thick. The thick mucus that develops is partially due to dry air and reduced nasal clearing during sleep time, leading to nasal stuffiness. Continue the routine of nasal saline spray before bedtime.

When using over-the-counter medications such as anti-histamines (for instance, Benadryl®), it's always good to check with your doctor first. Even though a prescription is not required, speak with your doctor regarding any potential side effects before starting any new medication. Anti-histamine medications may be helpful to 'dry up' the mucus and reduce nasal swelling, making it more comfortable for your child to sleep. They classically have a side effect of making people drowsy, but the newer ones occasionally have the reverse effect, and can make your child more excitable. When you first give your child an **anti-histamine**, try it at a time and place where either effect is acceptable to you — perhaps an early evening on a weekend night. You may be in for a wild child, or a snoozing one.

CHECK WITH YOUR DOCTOR BEFORE GIVING YOUR CHILD A COLD MEDICINE, EVEN IF IT DOES NOT REQUIRE A PRESCRIPTION

Decongestant medications containing **pseudoephedrine**, **ephedrine** or **phenylephrine** have been shown to have potential for serious side effects in young children. Several reports of life-threatening heart problems were seen in some children, prompting the FDA to issue warnings regarding the use of these medications in young children. Medications containing these drugs are not recommended for children under the age of four years. After the age of four years, they are approved for use, but it's always a good idea to check with your doctor first, to make sure that you are using the most appropriate medication for your child's particular symptoms.

My two-year old has a runny nose, and also started having a wet cough. He doesn't have a fever, and it doesn't seem to be slowing him down, but that cough sounds awful. What could be going on? Is there anything I could do?

Oftentimes a wet cough either follows or goes along with a runny nose. The reason for this is whatever you see coming out the front of your child's nose is also dripping down the back of his nose, into his throat. Toddlers are novices at nose blowing, so they tend to have more of the mucus from a cold dripping in all directions. This mucus drips slowly towards the voice box, and once enough of it accumulates, it triggers a cough reflex, which clears the mucus away. That mucus either gradually comes back to the voice box, triggering another cough, or it is swallowed. Swallowing mucus in and of itself is not bad, and usually doesn't cause any irritation in the stomach. After that, the cycle starts up all over again. Usually this cough becomes worse at night,

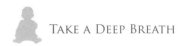

because as the mucus drips to the back, the swallowing muscles are not as active, which leads to accumulation of the mucus more towards the voice box, triggering more coughing and less swallowing. If your child has a runny nose and a wet cough, but seems happy, has a normal appetite, and no fever, it is likely a mild cold virus that is causing these symptoms. Most children with a stuffy nose will not feel 100% happy, simply due to the discomfort of having a stuffy nose. Saline is a die-hard helper for these situations. A couple of squirts, a few times per day, will help flush out some of the mucus. A humidifier in the bedroom also helps to loosen up the mucus, which tends to dry up and thicken at night. Cough medicine such as those containing **guaifenisen**, a medication that thins and loosens mucus, is not recommended for children under the age of four years. Medications containing anti-histamines such as **diphenhydramine** (such as Benadryl®) are also not recommended under the age of four years. **Oxymetazoline** (Afrin®) nasal spray may be used in limited quantities. Most pediatricians and ear, nose, and throat doctors recommend one to two sprays to each nostril, no more than two times per day for no more than two days (2-2-2). This spray acts to shrink down the swollen nasal lining, which, in turn, will lead to less mucus production and more airflow. But check with your doctor before giving this to your child.

This is a good time to start teaching your child, at least conceptually, how to blow his nose. However, it may be best to do so BEFORE he is sick, as it is easier to make a blowing motion when there is no mucus stuffing up the airflow. Show him the motion you make when you blow air out of his nose, and make it into a game. Hold an open tissue in front of his nostrils, and see if he can make it move. Fun! Close each nostril, and see if he can do it on each side. This may make nose blowing easier when the mucus starts flowing.

My three-year old has had a runny nose and a wet cough for over a week. When is it more than a cold?

Most colds run their course over three to seven days. But if your child does not seem to show any signs of improvement, or if she seems to be getting worse, the **viral** cold may be turning into a **bacterial** infection. Signs of a bacterial infection include green or yellow nasal discharge, foul breath, a wet cough for more than one week, fever, irritability, lethargy, and poor appetite. Your child does not need to have all of these signs, but any of these may be an indication that a bacterial infection is brewing. Many parents assume that if the mucus is yellow, it must be a bacterial infection. This is not necessarily the case, especially in kids who do not blow their noses well (or at all). The longer the mucus stays in the nose, the darker the color. While color change may be a sign of a bacterial infection, it may simply be due to the fact that the mucus is a bit stagnant. The difference between a viral infection and a bacterial infection, at least when it comes to colds, is that a viral infection is treated with 'supportive' measures such as humidification, saline, lots of fluids, and rest, while a bacterial infection needs all of these measures, in addition to **antibiotics**. Many bacterial infections begin as viral infections. Bacteria love to grow in the warm, moist, environments of swollen tissue and mucus that viruses create. If your child has a runny nose/wet cough with fever, decreased appetite, and low energy, give your doctor a call. She may want you to bring your child in to the office to evaluate her for the possibility of having a bacterial infection. If so, you will receive a prescription for antibiotics. However, don't be disappointed if your child does not receive antibiotics. Many viral infections can be similar to bacterial infections, and can even seem 'worse' than a bacterial infection.

What's the difference between a bad cold and a sinus infection? How can you tell them apart?

There is surprisingly no easy answer to this. Many people think that a green runny nose and a cough must mean a sinus infection. However, the sinuses are so tiny in young children, the largest one is no bigger than a small marble, and the smallest ones are each the size of a grape seed. If you get an **X-ray** (or even a **CT Scan**) on any young child with a cold, the sinuses will be filled with fluid, and, from a radiologic standpoint, will be considered to be 'sinusitis'. As a matter of fact, studies have shown that children who have CT Scans of the sinuses for reasons other than a cold (head or facial injury, brain tumors, etc) will have incidental signs of 'sinusitis' on the CT Scans, in the absence of any cold symptoms at all. It is for this reason that a true diagnosis of a sinus infection in a child must be made by evaluating the associated symptoms, which can include:

❖ Fever
❖ Green or yellow runny nose for more than two weeks

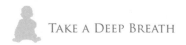

- ❖ Cough for more than two weeks
- ❖ Facial pressure or pain/irritability
- ❖ Foul-smelling breath
- ❖ Puffiness around the eyes
- ❖ Sticky drainage from the corners of the eyes
- ❖ X-ray evidence of sinusitis

A visit to the doctor will be needed to determine whether or not your child needs antibiotics for a sinus infection. Other measures, such as saline nasal spray, **oxymeta-zoline** (if your doctor says it's safe), humidification, drinking lots of liquids, **antihis-tamines**, **acetaminophen**, **ibuprofen**, and propping your child up with an extra pillow at night, will also help.

My four-year-old has had three sinus infections, and now she seems to have another one, with the exact symptoms as before. But when I called my doctor, he refused to call in a prescription without seeing my child. Is he being unreasonable?

No. While, in all likelihood, your child would do fine with the same, or a similar prescription for antibiotics as before, your doctor is being prudent, *and* reasonable, in asking you to bring your child in to be checked. There are a few reasons for this. First of all, one of the biggest problems that we have seen throughout the United States and many industrialized nations is antibiotic overuse. This has resulted in many bacterial infections being resistant to antibiotics, which has led to the need for much stronger antibiotics to fight what used to be 'routine' bacteria, as well as the need for higher and higher doses of these antibiotics to be effective. Young children are commonly receiving what used to be adult dosing for common bacterial infections. Why has this happened? First of all, most infections (including ear infections, throat infections, sinus infections, and tonsillitis) are viral. Even though this is the case, we have become an 'overprescribing' world, giving too many antibiotics unnecessarily, in an effort to prevent complications from the occasional bacterial infection. When millions of people receive antibiotics for years and years, over time, the 'stronger' or 'different' bacteria survive and grow. These bacteria, in turn, cause new infections, requiring newer and/or stronger antibiotics.

So, your doctor wants to check your child to see if she really does need antibiotics, and, if so, which one she needs, and, if so, what is really being treated. Perhaps this time she also has an ear infection, or maybe it's worse than before, and she has bronchitis or early pneumonia. Or, indeed, maybe it's just the same old sinus infection that never really cleared up from the last one. But have her checked first.

My preschooler is a lovely little princess, but lately she smells terrible. I can't seem to identify anything, except that the odor seems to be coming from her face. Her teeth are clean, I bathe her daily, she doesn't soil herself, and she doesn't seem sick. What am I missing?

I've had the most meticulous parents nearly drop off their child in my office to fix the smell. When in doubt, think pussy willows! Toddlers are fascinated with their bodies, but they have yet to learn that their noses are not pockets. Pussy willows are historically common items to stick up the nose — they are soft, fun to play with, and they fit! Items such as these (as well as any seeds, beans, beads, tissues) are often hidden by toddlers for who knows how long before any symptoms appear. And the symptom may be just that she smells bad! More often, she will have a runny nose 'on one side', or a stuffy nose 'on one side'. When you bring a child to a doctor and the mystery of the lodged — (fill in the blank) is discovered, you will of course ask your princess 'did you put — in your nose?'. The answer (and this goes for older kids too), will be one of three: a shrug, 'no', or 'my big brother did it'. Feel free to ask, but don't expect an answer of any value, especially as you, the doctor, and the nurse are ganging up in a mini-inquisition. Instead, gently but firmly explain to your princess (interestingly, girls are five times more likely than boys to stick things up their noses) that her royal nose is not a pocket, not a hiding place, and not a storage unit for toys, jewels, or snacks.

Most pediatricians, emergency room physicians, or ear, nose, and throat specialists will be able to remove a nasal object in the office, although they will likely need

GIRLS ARE FIVE TIMES MORE LIKELY TO PLACE OBJECTS IN THEIR NOSES THAN BOYS

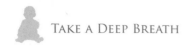

some assistance from a firm parent to hold their child still. Occasionally, if the object has become lodged to the point of being not visible, or if the nasal tissue is too swollen and irritated, your child may need to have a brief general anesthesia in an operating room to have the object safely removed.

I was changing the battery in my camera and I can't find the old one. I think my daughter stuck it up her nose. What do I do?

Bring her to a doctor, urgent care, or emergency room right away. This is serious. Disc batteries are more and more commonly used for electronic equipment, watches, cameras, and toys, but they are really dangerous to children. When these batteries are exposed to a warm, moist environment such as the inside of someone's nose, they begin to cause tissue damage within minutes or just a few hours. They leak a fluid that can permanently erode through tissues, and they also create an electrical current, resulting in even more damage. If a disc battery stays inside the nose for more than a few hours, it can cause permanent damage to the nose, by creating a permanent hole in the nasal **septum** (the center cartilage of the nose that separates the right side from the left, and also gives support to the tip of the nose), or it can cause an injury to the sinuses by damaging the nasal bones. As you know, disc batteries come in all sizes, and the small ones used for watches, cameras, and children's toys can easily fit in a small child's nose.

My four and a half-year-old has a runny nose, watery eyes, and sneezes all Spring and Fall. Can he have allergies?

Yes. Allergies can begin to be more clearly recognized as children are into the preschool years. Classic signs include:

❖ Clear runny nose (may or may not be stuffy)
❖ Watery eyes (sometimes the white part can turn red)
❖ Sneezing
❖ Generalized itchiness, even without a rash
❖ Puffiness or dark circles under the eyes (this occurs because nasal congestion can lead to congestion of the tear ducts, which, in turn causes the tissues around the eyes to swell and become a bit darker. It is also a result of overall facial congestion or 'puffiness', secondary to chronic nasal stuffiness and constant breathing through the mouth).

❖ A straight horizontal line of lighter skin (almost looks like a very fine scar) over the middle part of the nose (this is termed an 'allergic salute', as it develops from a child continually rubbing their nose in an upward direction due to itchiness or mucus — it appears as if they are 'saluting' their nose).

Indications that your child may have allergies also include the fact that his symptoms are seasonal. He may get 'sicker' during these seasons, as a child with allergies tends to have a baseline degree of nasal swelling and mucus, which may make them more predisposed to respiratory illnesses such as viral colds or bacterial sinusitis. Seasonal allergies are more likely 'outdoor' allergies, such as pollens, grasses, trees, or plants. Indoor allergies usually carry similar symptoms as outdoor allergies, but they last all year round. Substances that trigger indoor allergies include dust, dust mites, pets, feather pillows, and mold. Children with both indoor and outdoor allergies may improve when they travel, where they are less likely to be exposed to the allergens triggering their symptoms.

Your child can be tested for allergies at this age, and some specifics regarding what they are or are not allergic to can also be assessed. However, as your child still has a somewhat immature immune system, some of the testing may reveal 'negative' results, which may become 'positive' when they are a bit older (around the age of four or five years). Some allergy medications, including **antihistamines** and **nasal steroid sprays** are approved for use in children over the age of two years. Some of these (especially antihistamines) are sold over-the-counter, with no prescription required. However, check with your doctor before starting any medication for your child, even if it doesn't require a prescription.

My five-year-old seems stuffy all of the time. Even when he's not sick, he's congested. He has no signs of any sort of allergy. What else could it be?
Usually sometime between the age of two and six years, there is a period of growth of the **lymphoid tissue** of the face and neck. This tissue is often referred to as 'glands' or, more accurately, 'lymph nodes'. As a child's immune system matures, this tissue grows, with or without illness. One area of lymphoid tissue that grows in the back of the nose is the **adenoids**. While the word is plural, the adenoids are actually one 'area' of lymphoid tissue, located in the very back part of the nose, up behind the roof of the mouth. If you think of your head as an earth, the adenoids are at the core. One cannot see

147

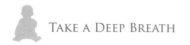

adenoids by looking in the mouth, nor by looking at the front part of the nose. When the adenoids grow, this growth can cause nasal symptoms such as stuffiness, congested speech (it sounds like he has a cold when he doesn't), runny nose, sinus infections, snoring, drooling, or 'mouth breathing' (your child always breathes through his mouth, when awake and asleep). So if adenoids enlarge, and a doctor can't see them, how do we know if they are the culprit? There are a few ways to assess adenoids: One is to pass a tiny fiberoptic camera (the width of a thin spaghetti strand) into the back of the nose. A few drops of anesthetic are placed into the nose before doing this. It is slightly uncomfortable, but usually lasts about thirty seconds or less. Another way to assess adenoid size is to obtain an X-ray of the soft tissues of the neck (one lateral, or profile view). This will give a great picture of what percent of the nasal airway is being blocked by adenoid tissue. Anything over 50% is considered to be enlarged adenoids.

If your doctor thinks that your child's nasal stuffiness is caused by enlarged adenoids, he may or may not recommend removal. This is a discussion you will have with your pediatrician, allergist (if allergies are also involved), and ear, nose, and throat specialist. Adenoid removal is usually recommended if the nasal symptoms are interfering significantly with day-to-day activities or nighttime sleep for your child. There is no clear-cut yes/no answer for this. It usually comes down to how detrimental the nasal stuffiness is for your child, and how big his adenoids are in relation to his nasal air passages. If you go ahead with adenoid surgery (adenoidectomy), it is, in almost all cases, a very well tolerated surgery, even for children as young as two years old. It is performed under general anesthesia, usually takes about fifteen minutes, most kids go home on the day of surgery, and most have a very mild (if any) sore throat for a few days after surgery. Most kids resume normal activities within a few days following adenoid removal. You will of course go over the details of your child's particular situation with your doctors, but in general, it is a relatively easy surgery for kids (and parents) to handle.

My five-year-old has a chronic stuffy nose. She doesn't have allergies, and doesn't have enlarged adenoids. But she is pretty uncomfortable, both day and night. Is there anything we can do?
Children (and adults) can develop an entity termed **vasomotor rhinitis**, which is essentially 'non-allergic stuffy nose'. The tissues of the nose become just as swollen

as they would in the setting of allergies, but all allergy testing is negative. Vasomotor rhinitis symptoms are similar to allergy symptoms — stuffy nose, congestion, occasional runny nose, and predisposition to more colds and sinus infections. Many prescription **Nasal steroid sprays,** such as Flonase®, Nasonex®, Veramyst® and Omnaris®, are safe medications in children over the age of two years. They are given once or twice per day (depending on your child's age), and work by shrinking the nasal tissues. They are not absorbed into the bloodstream as are inhaled steroids in nebulizers, so there is no concern for steroid side effects as when they are inhaled, taken by mouth or given as a shot. Nasal steroid sprays work only if they are used on a regular basis (daily), and it usually takes a week or two before you will start to see an effect. Most children tolerate them quite well. The mist is very fine, and not irritating to the tissues.

My child has a chronically stuffy nose. He does not have allergies.
We have tried nasal steroids for six months, antihistamine medications,
antibiotics for infections, and saline spray. His adenoids are normal.
Is there a last resort?

It could be that he has enlarged or swollen turbinates. The turbinates are the liners in each side of the nose. They are important for nasal function but can get in the way of breathing comfortably if they become too enlarged. There is a last resort to treat the turbinate swelling. When all medication options fail, there is a small procedure that can be performed, called **turbinate reduction**. This is a procedure whereby a small instrument is placed into the nose (under general anesthesia, if it is a child), and this instrument acts to shrink the **nasal turbinates**. We need our turbinates for nasal moisture and filtering of dust particles, which is why enlarged turbinates are shrunk but not removed. The procedure is very safe and takes about 15 minutes to complete, but it must be performed under general anesthesia, where your child is completely asleep. Most kids have minimal to no discomfort afterwards, and need to miss only a day or two of school or activities. It is so 'non-invasive', that adult turbinate reduction is often performed in a doctor's office, with some local anesthesia such as novacaine.

THE BIG PICTURE

Stuffy and runny noses are commonplace in the toddler group. Some parents describe their child as 'always stuffy' or 'always runny' for all or part of the calendar year. The vast majority of these children have mild, frequent colds that seem to either blend into one long cold, or overlap with one another, especially during the school year, which of course corresponds with the respiratory illness seasons. However, children who have recurrent acute illnesses beyond colds, or have nasal stuffiness to the point of interfering with their daytime functioning (which, at these ages translates to eating, sleeping, running, and playing), may need to be evaluated for possible triggers such as environmental allergies or adenoid enlargement. Children with nasal symptoms in one nostril need to be evaluated for a foreign object. Toddlers are renowned for sticking objects up their nose. Most objects are not call for alarm, but anytime you suspect that your child has placed a battery in his nose, call the doctor or go to an emergency room right away.

DON'T WORRY

If your child has recurrent (or even chronic) stuffy noses, but seems happy and active, sleeps comfortably, eats well, and is not coughing, there is very little to be concerned about. This is a very common issue in growing toddlers, especially if they either have an older sibling, or are involved in any sort of playgroup, daycare, or preschool environment. This is the time to emphasize the importance of good hygiene (especially hand washing and nose-blowing), and to teach your kids how 'cover your cough' and 'cover your sneeze' (into the crook of their arm, not onto their hand). These two techniques really cut down the spread of respiratory illnesses.

If your child gets a little too excited about nose blowing into tissues, and starts sticking them (and leaving them) up her nose, while they do need to be removed, it is nothing to panic over. Some kids make a habit of putting things up their noses. This is one to break early. And kids are quick at this age. Teach them that pants have pockets, but noses do not. If your toddler has nasal inclinations, keep her fingernails short. Nose picking starts at around this time, and, while it is a habit that needs to be broken, you don't want your child unnecessarily scratching her delicate nose in the habit-breaking process.

Chronic nasal stuffiness in the absence of a cold may be either due to environmental allergies, non-allergic nasal congestion, or enlarged adenoids. A specialist (allergist or ear, nose, and throat specialist) can help make this assessment. Intervention may or may not be necessary, depending on how mild or severe the nasal stuffiness is.

WORRY

If your child has nasal stuffiness to the point of having complete inability to breathe through his nose, he may need a more thorough and prompt evaluation for the source of the nasal blockage. While kids at this age (actually after the age of three or four months) can compensate well by breathing through their mouths, it's a pretty miserable existence to be unable to breathe through ones nose. Ask your doctor to check it out, or to refer you to a specialist.

If your child sticks a battery of any kind up her nose, or if you THINK your child MAY have stuck a battery up her nose, seek medical attention right away.

TO-DO LIST: STUFFY NOSE/RUNNY NOSE/SINUSITIS — FROM FRIENDS AND FOES

1. Expect some stuffy and runny noses during toddlerhood, especially during the fall and winter. They are not necessarily signs of severe illness.

2. Saline, saline, saline. For runny or stuffy noses, especially in the absence of illness, nasal saline, as a spray, drops, or irrigation, is the best treatment and prevention for runny noses.

3. If your child's runny nose goes from clear to yellow or green, and he is also coughing and has a fever, that is the time to give your doctor a call.

4. Check with your doctor before starting any medication for your child's runny or stuffy nose — even if a prescription is not required.

5. Teach your tot about nasal hygiene — noses are not pockets or hiding places.

6. Most objects placed into the nose do not require emergency attention, except for a battery of any kind. Batteries in the nose require immediate medical attention.

7. Objects left in the nose too long will lead to a foul smell. Beans placed in the nose will most likely sprout if left untouched.

8. By the age of three years, toddlers should begin to (or master) nose blowing. Practice by 'blowing' objects such as tissue paper when your child's nose is clear. Start by having her use both nostrils, then one at a time.

9. Most runny or stuffy noses do not necessitate antibiotics. Your doctor will help in deciding whether or not your child has a bacterial illness that requires antibiotic treatment.

10. If your child is always stuffy, it may not be due to a cold. It may be caused by environmental allergies, non-allergic stuffy nose, or enlarged adenoids. Your doctor can refer you to a specialist (allergist or ear, nose, and throat specialist) to make this assessment.

Sources for Stuffy-Nosed Toddlers:
www.entnet.org/healthinformation/coldremedies
www.entnet.org/healthinformation/pediatricsinusitis
www.entnet.org/healthinformation/allergicrhinitis

Chapter Sixteen
Snoring: What's That Noise?

Up to 85% of all young children snore at some point. So, snoring is in many ways a normal part of breathing patterns for young children. However, some types of snoring can be life-altering, even for young toddlers. This chapter will introduce what to look for and listen for in your snoring child, what snoring actually is, and what body parts are causing it. It will also present what snoring may do to the sleep cycles of young children, how it may impact your child's quality of sleep, and how it impacts the quality of their days.

Sleep apnea in children is less common than snoring, but it is now known to be more common than we thought years ago. Sleep apnea in children is part of a spectrum of disorders (known as 'obstructive sleep disorders' or 'sleep-disordered breathing'). This chapter will explain the differences in this spectrum of disorders, what the causes are, and what the possible treatments are. It will also describe what sleep apnea does to your child's sleep cycles and wake cycles on a daily and nightly basis.

My two-year-old has always snored a little, but over the last six months she sounds terrible every night. I can hear her from the next room, even with her door closed. Is this normal?

Most children, especially toddlers, will have some degree of snoring at some point. By definition, snoring is a noise caused by blockage at one of several possible parts of the airway: the nose, the back of the nose (or **nasopharynx**), the soft part of the roof of the mouth (**soft palate**), the back of the mouth, or the back of the tongue. During sleep, all of the muscles in the mouth and neck relax, and can lead the

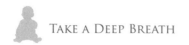
structures in the mouth or nose to hit up against each other and cause a snoring sound. It is because of this 'relaxed state' that snoring does not occur when kids are awake. They are better able to support the muscle structures, and breathe air around any possible blockage.

If a child snored as an infant and young toddler, and his snoring worsens with age, it is possible that some of the structures in the mouth and nose are growing out of proportion to the growth of his air passages. The most common cause for worsening of snoring in toddlers is enlargement of the **tonsils** and/or **adenoids**. The tonsils and adenoids are lymph nodes. The tonsils are located in the back of the mouth, one on each side, and the adenoids are located behind the roof of the mouth, behind the nose. You can look at the back of your child's mouth and see the tonsils directly. Adenoids (the word is plural, but it is actually one area of tissue), however, cannot be seen, as they are located above the palate. There is usually a normal period of growth of a child's lymph nodes between ages two and six years. If the tonsil and adenoid growth is significant, it may cause snoring. The reason why some children have this growth whereas others do not is not known, although it is thought to be in part due to genetic factors and/or low-grade infections (colds or coughs). The 'infections' theory, however, seems unlikely, as most kids with enlarged tonsils and adenoids do not have significant histories or sore throats, or even tonsillitis.

In answer to the question of whether an increase in snoring is normal or not, it depends on how severe the snoring problem is. Loud snoring in and of itself is not a concern, as long as the breathing pattern is 'regular' (in and out, without breaks or pauses), your child sleeps comfortably all night, and does not seem irritable during the day. Many parents can't tell if their child is sleeping well, or if the breathing pattern is 'regular' or not. In these cases, one option is to tape record (or video) a few minutes of his sleep, and have the pediatrician hear how it sounds. The 'gold standard' of identifying how severe a snoring problem is, is to have your doctor order a **sleep study**. A sleep study is an overnight test, either performed at a sleep laboratory or at your home (some sleep study companies can bring their equipment to your home). Monitors (stickers) are placed on your child's chest, head, and fingers, ideally after they have fallen asleep. These monitors measure how often your child snores, how this snoring affects his oxygen levels, and how often (if ever) your child has episodes of **apnea** (where they are trying to breathe but cant because of obstruction), and how long these episodes last. A physician trained in **Sleep Medicine** will interpret the test results, and determine whether or not your child has a significant sleep disorder or just has noisy breathing.

My three-year-old snores loudly. Sometimes he seems to gasp for air, hold his breath, and then take a big breath. He does this all night. What's going on?

'Breath-holding' during sleep is the most common sign of **sleep apnea**. Your child is trying to breathe, but his airway is blocked. When there is blockage, you will hear snoring, followed by silence, and then by a big gasp. This cycle keeps repeating. Here's what's happening: Your child tries to take a big breath, but something is in his way (usually big tonsils and adenoids, although your doctor needs to determine this for sure). When there is no air movement, the level of **carbon dioxide** (the gas we exhale) in the bloodstream goes up. Increased carbon dioxide in the blood sends a message to the breathing receptors in the brain. This message is: 'Wake up!'. The brain will 'wake up' from a deep sleep, and your child will 'wake up' and gasp for air. He will then (again) go back to sleep, and the apnea/carbon dioxide/wake/breathe cycle repeats. These 'mini wakenings' are not real 'waking up' in the conscious sense. They are just enough of a wakening to breathe, and to disrupt sleep. This is why both kids and adults with sleep apnea may think that they sleep all night, but are exhausted in the morning. Their brain has not had a good night's sleep. Many children with sleep apnea will tire more easily than their playmates. Alternatively, children with poor quality sleep can often be 'tired and wired'. Fatigue in young children can also be seen as hyperactivity. Any parent who has a nap-dependent toddler who misses a nap can easily describe their child running in circles at the end of a napless day. They certainly don't seem tired in the traditional sense, but they are.

If you think your child has sleep apnea (most kids with sleep apnea also have really loud snoring), you should let your doctor know. This isn't something that should wait until the next routine check-up. While it's usually not an emergency, it needs to be addressed. If your doctor sees that your child's tonsils and adenoids are enlarged, he will likely refer you to an ear, nose, and throat specialist for an evaluation.

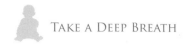

My four-year-old needs to have his tonsils and adenoids out. What do I need to know?

The vast majority of kids who get their tonsils and adenoids out these days are having this procedure done because of breathing problems during sleep (loud snoring, poor quality sleep, or sleep apnea). Most parents seek help because they are somewhat worried about their child's breathing at night. Your doctor will go over the details of what to expect, but here are some general guidelines:

1. Most kids go home after tonsil and adenoid surgery. But if your child is quite young (some institutions recommend under three years, some under two years) or has severe sleep apnea, it may be recommended that he stays overnight in the hospital.

2. Tonsil and adenoid surgery takes about 15 to 45 minutes, and it is performed under **general anesthesia** (kids are completely asleep).

3. There are over 100 methods of performing the surgery. There is no 'best technique'. It is important to find the surgeon you like best and to let her decide what technique she prefers the most.

4. It hurts after tonsillectomy, although it is less painful than it was in the past.

5. Most kids still need several days of pain medicine and reduced activity.

6. Most kids still need several days of ice cream and popsicles (although sometimes these are just for the 'treat' effect, and not because they cannot eat regular food).

7. In many kids, the breathing at night gets better right away. Sometimes there is some swelling of the tissues where the tonsils and adenoids once were, leading to temporary noisy breathing before improvement.

TONSILLECTOMY AND ADENOIDECTOMY IS STILL ONE OF THE MOST COMMON SURGERIES PERFOMED IN CHILDREN

8. As with all surgeries, there are certain risks in tonsil and adenoid surgery. The most common risks of tonsil surgery are bleeding, dehydration (if your child refuses to eat or drink afterwards), and deterioration of breathing problems. Go over the specifics with your doctor.

9. The majority of kids are completely better by seven to 14 days after surgery.

10. One of the most common complaints I get from parents of kids who've had tonsil and adenoid surgery is that they cant hear their child breathe at night anymore — it's too quiet!

My 20-month-old snores pretty loudly, and breathes with her mouth open all day. She sounds like she has a cold when she doesn't. Her doctor said that her tonsils are small. What else can it be?

Toddlers can have significant sleep problems (snoring, or even sleep apnea) even with normal tonsils. In this setting, the **adenoids** alone may be the culprit. Because the adenoids are not seen directly when looking in the nose or mouth, they need to be visualized differently. One option is to place a tiny fiberoptic camera (the width and texture of an undercooked spaghetti strand) into the back of the nose (after applying some topical numbing drops). The adenoids are located about three inches behind the front part of the nose, so the camera needs to get back there in order for the doctor to get a good look. The other method is to obtain an X-ray of the back of the nose. This is a plain X-ray (not a CT scan), and is one view in profile (similar to sinus X-rays, but from a different angle). These X-rays will give an image of the size of the adenoid tissue in relation to the air passage. It is 'normal' for a toddler to have a moderate amount of adenoid tissue, but if it is blocking the nasal air passage, it may be the explanation for your child's breathing problems. In the setting of large adenoids and small tonsils, your doctor may recommend that your child have his adenoids (and not tonsils) removed. This is a similar surgical procedure to the tonsil and adenoid surgery, but the recovery is much easier. This is because the adenoids are located behind the roof of the mouth, and the removal site is not exposed to food or air after the surgery. If you look into a child's mouth after adenoid surgery, it will look the same as it did before.

My almost three-year-old has loud snoring. Her doctor told me that she has normal adenoids and tonsils, and they are not blocking her airway. What else could be going on?

If your child snores, but has normal tonsils and adenoids (they are not blocking the air passages), one possibility is that the nasal passages are blocked. Inside the nasal passages are tissues called **turbinates**. Everyone has three sets of

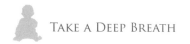

turbinates (inferior, middle, and superior), one set in each nostril. The inferior turbinates are most responsible for breathing issues. These can become swollen in both children and adults, either from environmental allergies (termed **allergic rhinitis**), or as a non-allergic local swelling (**non-allergic rhinitis, or vasomotor rhinitis**). Some children with nasal stuffiness and snoring, in the absence of enlarged tonsils and adenoids, may have enlarged turbinates. These can be seen directly during an examination by your pediatrician. It is often recommended for your child to be tested for allergies. If they have environmental allergies (food allergies do not typically cause nasal congestion), allergy treatment, either in the form of environmental modification (removing an allergen, if possible), or allergy medications, may help to reduce the size of the swollen turbinates. This can often reduce nasal congestion/snoring caused by enlarged turbinates. If your child does not have allergies, local measures to reduce nasal swelling may be recommended, such as topical nasal steroid sprays. Very rarely, if your child has severely enlarged turbinates with snoring, there are surgical procedures (**turbinate reduction**) which can be performed to reduce turbinate swelling. These are usually a reserved for those who have severe symptoms of nasal congestion despite a trial of medical therapies.

My five-year-old has always snored. It hasn't really affected his daily life, but his teachers are raising some concerns about his ability to focus, and they are concerned about his readiness for kindergarten.

Sometimes the first person to raise parents' awareness of a sleep disorder is a teacher. Even low-level snoring can be a sign of a sleep disorder, indicating that your child may not be getting the restful sleep you think he is getting. He may be in bed 'asleep' for ten hours each night, but he may be getting only six or seven hours of actual quality sleep. Teachers may notice that 'five-year-old behavior' is not being achieved, and they may raise some red flags of concern. A three- or four-year-old who is not getting quality sleep may act 'wild', 'out of control', 'volatile', or 'disruptive' both at home and at school. Sounds pretty typical, so most will just chalk it up to age and immaturity. But when the five-year birthday rolls around, a certain degree of civility is expected. Kids need to sit still for longer periods of time, focus longer, stay on task longer, push themselves in challenging tasks longer, be more patient, and learn to

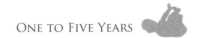

> **MOST CHILDREN WHO HAVE THEIR TONSILS AND ADENOIDS REMOVED ARE HAVING THE SURGERY TO IMPROVE BREATHING DURING SLEEP, AND TO IMPROVE SLEEP QUALITY.**

control impulses. In the setting of normal sleep, this is not an easy task, let alone in the setting of sleep deprivation. But again, he may not be an 'up all night' child. He, and you, may think he sleeps all night. But if you are starting to get calls from the teacher about focus issues or behavioral concerns, check on your child's sleep. Sleep disorders are not the cause of entities such as **Attention Deficit Hyperactivity Disorder (ADHD)**, but they certainly can (1) appear similar in terms of behavioral issues and/or (2) exacerbate behaviors associated with ADHD. Most ADHD specialists have become more aware of the link between sleep quality and ADHD manifestations, and will obtain a good history of your child's sleep quality if ADHD is being investigated. Parents must be aware that fixing a sleep disorder will not 'cure' ADHD. But it can lessen the symptoms, if they have been magnified by poor sleep quality.

THE BIG PICTURE

Children in the toddler years will usually have some degree of snoring at some point during these years. Some will only snore when they are sick, and some will snore all the time. Snoring in and of itself implies that there is some sort of 'obstruction' or 'blockage' somewhere in the air passages between the nose and the back of the mouth. The airflow is experiencing 'turbulence'. A little turbulence is fine (just as it is in air travel), but severe 'turbulence', will disrupt air travel, just as it will disrupt air flow. When snoring is heard, but there is 'regular' in and out breathing, with no gasping, coughing, choking sounds, or periods of pauses in breathing, it is usually nothing to be too concerned about. However, when snoring is very loud, and is associated with restless sleep, struggling to breathe, gasping, coughing, choking, or pauses in breathing, it needs to be addressed with your doctor. Many doctors do not routinely ask about snoring during regular check-ups, so don't hesitate to raise the issue if you are concerned. In the first year, the focus is on getting your baby to sleep through the night. When that mission is accomplished, the sleep quality question may fall by the wayside. So if your doctor doesn't ask about *how* your child is sleeping, and you think you hear some noise during sleep, bring it up during a visit, or call your doctor if there is no visit scheduled in the near future.

Poor sleep in older toddlers and preschoolers may actually be more obvious in the waking hours than in the sleeping hours themselves. Snoring or sleep apnea results in a bad night's sleep, night after night. This, in turn, leads to difficult days, poor focus, poor learning, and poor behavior. How easy would it be for you to, say, learn to play violin (assuming you didn't already play) after three months of sleep deprivation? That's how a five-year-old feels about learning to sit still and listen after countless nights of sleep-disordered breathing. If behavior issues are being raised at school, look into your child's sleep quality. Snoring? Tossing and turning? Occasional breaks in his breathing pattern? Let your doctor know about it.

DON'T WORRY

If your child has occasional snoring, but seems to have a regular 'in and out' pattern to her breathing, there is little to be concerned about. You may notice that there is very light snoring at some hours of the night, and other times when there is no snoring at all. This is likely because different stages of sleep are 'deeper', where the muscles are more relaxed, leading to more snoring. You may also notice that your child snores more when she has a cold. As long as the snoring subsides or improves when she is well, there is little to worry about. If your child sleeps soundly, seems comfortable, and is at ease during the day, a little snoring is part of the normal, varied sleep pattern.

WORRY

If your toddler has severe snoring, with loud enough breathing to hear in the next room (or even the next floor), has periods of silence followed by a big gasp for air, or seems to be struggling to breathe during sleep (you may see his chest move up and down, but no breathing occurring for several seconds at a time), your toddler may have a form of **obstructive sleep apnea.** This is not normal in children, just as it is not normal in adults. It can have both short- and long-term health impacts, including daytime fatigue, irritability, and poor attention. It can also have more severe health impacts. Chronic strain on the lungs from sleep apnea can lead to high blood pressure, heart disease, and lung disease. Disruption in the quality of sleep can impact both physical growth as well as brain development. If you think your child has a sleep problem, let your doctor know right away. It may not be something that is being asked during check-ups. There are many options for treating sleep problems in children. The earlier the treatment, the less likely that any long-term effects will occur.

TO-DO LIST: SNORING: WHAT'S THAT NOISE?

1. Just because your child sleeps through the night does not mean that she is a perfect sleeper. Check on her periodically to see how her breathing pattern looks and sounds.

2. Your child should breathe through her nose, when she is awake as well as during sleep. If she is a mouth breather at night, she may have a mild form of snoring or sleep apnea.

3. Mild snoring is normal in children. Loud snoring is not.

4. If your child has loud snoring, with periods of gasping, pauses in breathing, coughing, or choking, let your doctor know right away.

5. If your child is in daycare, ask his daycare provider if he snores during naps. Experienced daycare providers are often the 'first line' players in detecting sleep apnea in young children — after all, they are awake when your child is not!

6. Snoring in children is not the same as snoring in adults. Just because your spouse snores does not make it ok for your child to snore.

7. You can do a 'mini home sleep study'. Video tape or audio tape your child at a time when you hear the snoring. Bring the finished product to your doctor's office.

8. Make sure the batteries on your device are charged before your visit. Countless parents have come to see me, eager to show me a perfect example of a video of

sleep apnea for their child — they bring the smart phone or camera right up to me, and lo and behold — battery is dead.

9. Most causes of sleep disorders in children are curable, either by medical or surgical therapies. The most common cause of obstructive sleep apnea in children is enlarged tonsils and adenoids. Most of the 500,000 children per year in the United States who have their tonsils and adenoids removed have this procedure to treat sleep problems, not tonsillitis or sore throats.

Sources for Snoring: What's that Noise?

www.sciencedaily.com/releases/2003 ("Snoring May Increase Risk of Learning Problems in Some Children")

www.sciencedaily.com/releases/2004 ("Breathing Problems During Sleep May Affect Mental Development in Infants and Young Children")

www.sciencedaily.com/releases/2007 ("Sleep Disorders Can Impair Children's IQ's As Much As Lead Exposure")

Chapter Seventeen

Choking Hazards: What is Safe to Eat?

In the United States, one child dies every five days from a food choking accident, and over 10,000 children visit emergency rooms each year for food choking events. These are startling figures, especially since there are no established guidelines regarding safety of various foods at different ages. The majority of children who suffer from choking events are usually between 10 and 36 months, but older children can also have choking episodes. This chapter will give some 'unpublished' yet important food safety guidelines, based on my experience, to minimize choking accidents for your child.

These are the years when your child gains more and more independence from you. Many children are in full-time daycare or preschool before the age of three years, and are oftentimes exposed to older children in these settings. Food that your child receives by well-meaning adults or older children may not be in your control. It is astounding how little is known by even the most experienced and knowledgeable caregivers about food choking risks, and many well-established daycares and preschools routinely provide unsafe food to young children. In this situation, education is the best method of prevention. Public awareness of food safety is in its own infancy. Hopefully, in time, food safety will become as second nature as car seats and sunscreen.

My two-year-old was invited to a birthday party where popcorn was served as one of the snacks. Is this ok?
While popcorn is truly a 'fun' food of childhood, both in the preparing as well as in the eating, I do not recommend popcorn for toddlers under the age of four years.

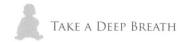

The main risk involves the sharp-edged, irregularly popped kernels. These pieces can become lodged in the back part of a young child's throat and get stuck, unable to be removed. Barely popped or completely unpopped popcorn kernels, which, as adults, we may look forward to at the bottom of the popcorn bowl, are extremely dangerous for young children. Kids can't bite into these, and these firm kernels can easily get accidentally passed into the windpipe. Popcorn alternatives that dissolve more readily, such as Pirates Booty®, cheese puffs, or even Cheetos® are much safer in this age group.

I went to the movies with my three-year-old, his best pal, and his best pal's mom. They bought a big bag of popcorn for all of us to share during the movie. How do I tell my child it is not safe, and tell the mom and her son as well?

This is a tough one. It will bring you back to the worst peer-pressured issues of high school: 'Everyone else is doing it, why cant I?' Ideally, this discussion can come up before you go to a movie theater, where popcorn is the most popular item consumed. But I would stand firm on this. When your child's safety is at issue, it is not a time to cave in to such pressure, even if it means splurging on an extra-special, yet safe, treat for both kids — ice cream, soft pretzels, even a sweet drink to diffuse some of the tears. Explain that popcorn is 'grown-up' food, or 'REALLY big kid' food, but there are plenty of other great kid foods that they can enjoy. Hopefully your friend will understand and be on your side. She may argue 'but he always eats popcorn!', but gently explain the risks of young children choking, especially in a dark movie theater. If she persists, you can quietly tell her that a young child died of choking on popcorn while in a noisy movie theater a few years back. Nobody saw or heard the child choking until it was too late. Unfortunately, this is a true story.

My son's pediatrician gives out lollypops in the office. Are these ok for toddlers?

In general, I recommend steering clear of any candy before the age of three years. However, it is hard to rationalize this, when our nation's top pediatric specialists are doling out the goods, right before these tots head to their cars. If you must give your child a lollypop, by all means do not let him eat in the car, nor while he is running in circles in the waiting room, listening to the screams of others receiving their vaccines. Lolly eating is a stationary activity. The least dangerous kinds are the ones that are flat circles (like a mini-pancake). Many of these will have a stick that is shaped as a loop, minimizing lolly stick injuries. The most dangerous kinds are spherical. These can be easily pulled off the stick, inhaled, and become lodged at the top of the airway. Not good, and poor form on the doctor's part if it happens in his waiting room. Teach kids early on that lollies are for licking — not for biting or pulling off of their sticks. If you know in advance that your doctor's office has treats which are not safe for your child, perhaps decide together with your child, on a great (reasonable) treat that he can have after his visit. Bring it with you to the visit. He will need it right away, especially if he can't have the treat that's offered in the office. Also consider gently, and delicately, mentioning to your doctor and/or her staff that spherical lollypops are choking hazards for young children, and that perhaps the office can consider altering the treat choices.

Can I give my three-year-old gum to chew?
While the old wives tale that swallowed gum stays in the stomach for seven years is untrue, gum is not safe for toddlers. Not only can it damage their teeth and jaw muscles, it poses a choking risk.

What about chips in this age group?
While they are not the healthiest of choices, chips can be eaten by older toddlers (over two years) if supervised by an adult. The main concerns about chips are the sharp edges that can poke the back of the throat if not adequately chewed (unlikely to cause any real damage, except some irritation), as well as large pieces causing a slight choking risk. Start with softer consistency chips such as thin potato chips before advancing to the triangular tortilla chips, and always remember to have your child seated while eating.

When can my child start eating peanut butter?
While all nuts and seeds should be reserved for older school children, nut butters (peanut butter, almond butter, soy butter, cashew butter) can be introduced between the age of two and three years. Many pediatricians feel that waiting

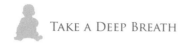

longer may reduce the risk of nut allergy, and that almond and soy are less aller-genic, and therefore recommend starting with these. From a breathing standpoint, the riskiest issue is that a large portion of any of the nut butters can get stuck at the back of the throat. After you clarify when nut butters could be given to your child, make sure that whichever one you choose is spread thinly on a soft cracker or a piece of bread. Eating spoonfuls of peanut butter straight from the jar is not recommended at this age, and start with smoother varieties, not chunky.

Can my toddler eat hotdogs?

For many reasons, kids love hotdogs. And for many different reasons, so do parents. For the kids, these are fun, tasty, salty foods that are easy to eat. For parents, they are easy to prepare, and they are foods with a semblance of nutritional value that kids will actually eat. They have a modicum of protein, and some versions such as 'low-fat', 'low-sodium', 'organic', 'kosher', 'vegetarian', or 'turkey' can actually pull off being somewhat healthy. But because they are a pre-formed tubular food, they can fit perfectly into a small child's air passage, usually at the back of the throat. When cut into penny-shaped discs, they can also lodge in the back of the throat. The safest way for toddlers to eat hotdogs is to cut the dog lengthwise in half, and then cut slices, making either half-moon discs or quarter moon wedges. A little less 'fun', but a lot safer. By age four or five, most kids will have learned to sit while they eat, and, if they do so, can eat a hotdog in its bun.

Can my four-year-old eat nuts?

Before age four, I don't think that any kid should eat any kind of nuts. After four, it really depends on the child. If you have an especially cooperative one, who can really sit still when she eats, 'softer' nuts such as walnuts and cashews are pretty reasonable. Whole almonds are a little tougher, as are peanuts. As with most new foods, gradually introduce them, and start with small pieces, to see if your child likes the taste and can handle the consistency.

Can my five-year-old chew gum?

Yes. Sugarless, if at all possible. But not while running around.

If my child chokes on a piece of food, is giving CPR the same as for an infant?

CPR for toddlers and older children is slightly different than CPR for infants. If your child chokes on a foreign object, whether it is some food or a toy, first assess whether or not he is crying or coughing. Crying and coughing are signs that your child's airway is not blocked. Let him try to clear the object on his own. If he has choked, and is not able to make any sound, the object is blocking his airway. First attempt the **Heimlich maneuver**. To perform this, stand behind your child, and wrap your arms around him, so that your grasped hands are just above his belly button. Give five quick thrusts, inward and upward, in an attempt to help him dislodge the object. If he begins coughing or crying, the object may be partially or completely dislodged out. Do not continue the maneuver, but see if he can clear it on his own. If he continues to be unable to make a sound, and is not breathing, begin CPR. If you are with someone, have them call 911. If you are alone with your child, perform CPR for two minutes, then call 911 and resume CPR after the phone call.

❖ Check your child's mouth for the object. If you can see it, remove it. If you cannot see it, give two breaths. Cover your child's mouth with your mouth and pinch his nose closed with your fingers before giving the breath. Remember, your child's lungs are smaller than yours, so small breaths are adequate.

❖ If your child does not begin breathing or coughing, place the heel of one hand in the middle of your child's breastbone, between his nipples. Push down about two inches, and then let the chest come back up. Do this 30 times, at the rate of about two compressions per second.

❖ Give two breaths again if he has not started breathing. Repeat the chest compression cycle. Continue this, alternating between breaths and chest compressions until help arrives.

❖ Even if your child resumes breathing, you still need to call 911 if CPR was needed.

THE BIG PICTURE

A few years back, I gave a talk at my daughter's preschool about food choking risks. One mother looked at me angrily, and asked "So what in the world can I feed my kid? You've left me no options! And while I'm at it, what in the world do you feed yours?" While many of the recommendations for food safety seem draconian or harsh, it really is not that bad. The vast majority of foods that we as adults eat are safe for young toddlers, however, many of the 'fun' kid foods, such as candy, gum, and popcorn, are not. While the risky foods are best to be avoided, what is most important is that your child eats under adult supervision, and that she does so when sitting down. The majority of food-choking accidents occur in the home, while the child is eating unattended or eating while running around.

DON'T WORRY

If you feel that you are subject to peer pressure on behalf of your toddler, do not worry, and do not cave. Your child will be offered foods from well-meaning adults (usually relatives or friends) which you know are not safe, and you will need to make an executive decision to refuse on your eager child's behalf. Expect some sneers from the adults, and tears from your child, but by all means do not worry. You are making the right decision! No, your two-year-old cannot have cashews, even though your family traditions include cashews at every family gathering. 'But you ate cashews at Johnny's age!' your aunt will cackle. ('and I didn't wear seatbelts', you will mutter under your breath). If you have the opportunity, and a somewhat receptive audience, feel free to give a well-deserved information session on the risks of food-choking in children. You may save someone else's child in the process.

WORRY

If your child is eating any sort of food, 'safe' or 'unsafe' and has a choking episode, it warrants medical attention, even if she seems fine right afterwards. If she seems PERFECT, at least give your doctor a call, to review signs to watch out for (more coughing, any wheezing sounds, breathing trouble, or vomiting may signal that there is a remnant of food stuck in your child's air passage). If your child has a sudden choking episode on a large food object, such as a spherical lollipop or a nut, begin with back thrusts and the **Heimlich maneuver** (for children over 12 months). The Heimlich maneuver is a method of releasing an object that is lodged in the upper air passages. It is performed by standing behind the choking victim, 'hugging' them just below the rib cage, and producing multiple brief tugs, upward and inward from the top of the stomach towards the ribs. Very often, this has been shown to be a successful method of dislodging an object, in both children and adults. If your child continues to choke and is not breathing, call 911 and begin CPR.

TO-DO LIST: CHOKING HAZARDS: WHAT IS SAFE TO EAT?

1. When in doubt, wait. Ask your pediatrician. Or check the American Academy of Pediatrics website (www.aap.org). There is a section on food safety.

2. Start slowly when advancing new foods with your toddler, especially if you are introducing new textures.

3. Nuts, hard candy, and gum should not be given to children under the age of three years.

4. Raw fruits and vegetables should be cut in very thin strips (not cubes) until kids are three to four years.

5. Fruits with skins, such as apples or grapes, should be peeled until children are three years old.

6. Grapes should be peeled, and then cut into smaller pieces until the age of three years.

7. Check with your pediatrician regarding the recommended age to begin 'nut butters' such as almond butter, cashew butter, soy butter, and peanut butter. Some recommend age two years, some three or even four years. Regardless of the age, remember to spread it thinly on bread or a soft cracker. No big spoonfuls of nut butter until college! The thick paste can lodge at the back of the throat.

8. No popcorn for toddlers under the age of four years.

9. Hotdogs need to be cut lengthwise and then in slices again, to create either 'half-moon' or 'quarter-moon' shapes. After age four, hotdogs in a bun are just fine.

Sources for Choking Hazards:

www.aap.org

www.cpsc.org

Chapter Eighteen

Hoarseness in Toddlers and Preschoolers: Shhhhh!

With the onset of talking may come loud talking, louder talking, and even yelling and screaming. The latter is seen especially in children of large families. Very commonly the youngest child, vying most for attention, is the most hoarse. **Hoarseness**, or a roughness in the voice, may come on suddenly, or last for months on end (chronic hoarseness). This chapter will reveal causes and possible treatments for sudden voice changes and chronic voice changes. The most common cause in this group is an entity called '**screamer's nodules**' from voice overuse and strain. However, rare chronic diseases of childhood may begin with hoarseness. Chronic hoarseness (greater than one month) in your child needs medical attention.

My 22-month-old has always had a rough, 'gravelly' voice. She is healthy, and she never loses her voice or has trouble breathing. I actually think it's cute. Do I need to get her checked?
In all likelihood, this is your daughter's voice, and there is probably nothing really 'wrong' with it. Children have 'rough' or 'deep' voices during infancy and childhood for several reasons — one possibility is that it is simply the pitch that her vocal cords produce, without any actual abnormality in the structure or function. Another possible reason is that your child has become accustomed to straining her voice, either by crying or yelling. This leads to chronic swelling of the tissues of the voice box, leading to a rough quality to the voice. There are also other possible causes, such as **gastroesophageal reflux**, where the acid that comes up from the esophagus and

stomach can cause irritation and swelling in the voice box. Lastly, children can develop growths on the vocal cords, leading to hoarseness.

IF YOUR CHILD IS HOARSE FOR MORE THAN ONE MONTH, LET YOUR DOCTOR KNOW

It is a good idea, even if your child is healthy, to have her voice checked out by a specialist (ear, nose, and throat) if she has been hoarse for a long time. They may take a tiny camera, the width of a spaghetti strand, and look at her vocal cords in the office. Before they would do this, they will give your child a few drops of numbing medication (**lidocaine**) into her nose. They will then place the camera into her nose. When it gets to the back of her nose, the doctor can get a 'bird's eye' view of all of the structures of the voice box, checking for movement of the vocal cords, redness, swelling, or any growths. The procedure is slightly uncomfortable (although less so after the numbing drops), but usually takes under one minute to complete.

My four-year-old son has been hoarse for six months, and now is making some wheezing sounds at night. I took him to a specialist who diagnosed him with papillomas. What are these?

Papillomas are small 'warts' that can grow on the vocal cords, even in young children. They are caused by the **human papillomavirus (HPV)** — the same virus that causes warts elsewhere in the body, including the genital areas. HPV can be transmitted from mom to baby while mom is pregnant, and the fetus can develop the same HPV infection seen in genital warts, but in children these appear on the voice box. Papillomas in the voice box are relatively rare (approximately 2500 children are diagnosed each year in the United States), but it is a problem that needs to be taken very seriously. Most children develop gradually worsening hoarseness, and because the growths may go untreated, unrecognized growth of papillomas can lead to breathing difficulties such as wheezing or complete loss of breathing function. Many children with papillomas are diagnosed with asthma, due to the wheezing sound the vocal cords can make, interfering with the child's ability to make a clear sound.

Eventually they may lose their voice completely, being only able to whisper. This is not asthma. Asthma does not cause hoarseness. A hoarse child, while he may also have asthma, needs to have his vocal cords looked at. Papillomas are one of the most commonly missed disorders in young children. Average delay in symptom onset to diagnosis is one to two years. Catching this disease in its earliest stages can be life-saving.

While there is no 'cure' for papillomas, there are many treatments available to keep the growths at bay, which you can discuss with your specialist (every major medical center has different treatment protocols). But you need to know that it will not be a 'one-time' treatment, and multiple treatments will be needed. The medical term for papillomas in the voice box is **recurrent respiratory papillomatosis (RRP).** As the name states, the disease is a 'recurrent' one, which needs to be followed quite closely. There is, to date, no 'best' or 'right' treatment, but it is important to stick with the treatment regimen recommended by your doctor. Treatment does involve trips to the operating room, either to remove the papillomas, and/or to administer medications to prevent them from growing back quickly. The surgeries are performed through telescopes looking into your child's mouth, without having cuts on the outside skin. The majority of children with papillomas 'grow out of it' by puberty. However, the severity of the disease differs in every individual, and every child with papillomas has a different degree of the disease.

If your child is diagnosed with RRP, there are support groups, both online and in person, which are very helpful. The RRP foundation is a wonderful source of information and guidance for families of children with RRP (www.rrpf.org).

How did my child get RRP? From daycare? From not washing his hands?

RRP is caused by HPV (human papillomavirus). This virus is transmitted from the mother's body to the baby. This is called 'maternal transmission' or 'vertical transmission'. Many mothers will report that they have had no history of genital warts, no abnormal pap smears, and no history of HPV. While this may be the case, over 50% of women carry HPV, and can transmit it to their baby. On the other hand, this does not mean that 50% of babies will develop HPV. A very small percentage of children develop this, but it is from maternal transmission. Many moms, upon hearing this, feel very guilty, that they 'gave' their child this disease. Again, a large percentage of

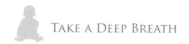

the population has this virus, but relatively few develop any signs or symptoms, nor is the virus always transmitted to the baby. Unfortunately, there was no way of preventing the transmission by any medical treatment given to mom during pregnancy. On the other hand, transmission of HIV (human immunodeficiency virus), can now be nearly 100% blocked if mom is treated with anti-viral medications during pregnancy. Perhaps, in the future, this may also be the case for prevention of HPV transmission.

My two-year-old has RRP, but I want more children. What are the chances of them having RRP? Would a Cesarian section prevent transmission of the virus?

RRP is seen almost exclusively in first-born children, even if mom continues to have active HPV infection. It is extremely unlikely that a second or subsequent children will have RRP. C-section has not been shown to prevent transmission of HPV, so a vaginal delivery is a reasonable option for second or third children.

Can I be tested for HPV? What about my spouse?

Yes. Pap smears can now include a test for HPV. Men can be tested via urethral swab. But, again, being HPV + does not necessarily mean, by any means, that your child will definitely have HPV. Millions and millions of people are HPV positive, while only a few thousand children develop growths from the virus. It is not known why only some children who are exposed go on to develop RRP.

Will the " Cervical Cancer Vaccine" prevent RRP in children?

While there remains much controversy surrounding this relatively new vaccine, it is indeed possible that if the next generation 'wipes out' this virus, we may no longer be transmitting it to our children. The theory behind this is that a large percentage of cervical cancer in women originates from an HPV infection. If HPV is eradicated in women and men, perhaps transmission to children can be eradicated as well. However, there are many 'strains' (or 'subtypes') of this virus, just as there are many 'strains' of the cold virus or the flu virus. The vaccine only prevents growth of some of the strains, not all. There is much research to be done in the field of HPV, cervical cancer prevention, as well as RRP.

My three-year-old seems to get hoarse at the end of each day, but his voice seems fine each morning. What could be going on?

Toddlers have difficulty in self-regulation when it comes to just about everything. No toddler will say "I'm tired, I think I need a nap", or "I'm full — I don't want another cookie". They follow suit when it comes to their voice. There is no 'inside voice' or 'outside voice' to them. There is just their 'voice', which for many needs to be used as loudly as possible. Most three–year–olds are in environments with many other three-year-olds for most of the day, and the one with the loudest voice is heard the best. So, your sweet son may spend the early morning hours serenely chatting with you, your spouse, and perhaps a sibling or two, but by mid-morning, he becomes immersed in a lion's den of like minds. They yell with excitement, squeal with enthusiasm, laugh with abandon. It is all so wonderful, the unhindered minds of young, eager children. But many will come home hoarse at the end of each day. They have strained themselves, including their voice box. When continuous force and effort is made on the fragile tissues of the vocal cords, these tissues become swollen, leading to a rough quality to the voice. In most cases, the 12 to 20 hours of home and rest will give the cords time to 'heal' each day.

My five-year-old has been hoarse for the last year.

If the yelling and loudness continues at home (very commonly in homes with many siblings, where the 'preschool scene' continues), the voice box does not have time to heal at the end of each day of activity. This may lead to chronic hoarseness — throughout the day, into the evening, as well as in the early morning hours. Some kids even 'lose' their voice at the end of each day. What's happening is that the swelling is firming up into little 'calluses' or 'nodules'. These nodules are tiny bumps on the vocal cords (usually one tiny bump on each cord, sitting directly opposite from the other side). Normally during speech, the vocal cords come together and make a smooth, slippery vibration, creating sound of a clear speech or song. When there is a tiny bump (even as small as 1 or 2 millimeters) on each one, the vocal cords cannot come together in a smooth fashion. Each time they do, a tiny bit of air sneaks up around them, creating the 'breathiness' that you hear when someone is hoarse.

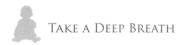

My son's hoarseness sounds kind of cute. Do I need to get rid of it?

Yes, it can sound cute, and yes, you need to get rid of it. Not that it is particularly dangerous, but those little tiny bumps can grow, leading to chronic hoarseness that will be very difficult to treat. Just as calluses develop from blisters if you wear the wrong shoes, and those calluses will continue to grow if you continue wearing those shoes, **vocal nodules** (affectionately known as 'screamer's nodules) can grow as well. Your child's vocal cords need 'new shoes'. Most children over three will be able to benefit from **voice therapy.** This is very similar to speech therapy, however, a voice therapist focuses on loudness control and breath control, as opposed to articulation or enunciation. Some three-year-olds will be able to focus enough to learn some voice techniques, especially if you can find a particularly patient voice therapist with experience in treating young children (we are lucky enough to have two in our practice). Most of the work, however, is done at home, not with the therapist. The voice therapist will give you as a parent, and you as a family, techniques in modulating loudness levels and vocal strain. Oftentimes the voice therapist ends up giving a mini voice therapy session to the parents, who are quite often contributors to the loudness factor.

My eighteen-month old has had croup several times. She has had a mild cold for a few days, but tonight before bedtime she sounded hoarse.

Be prepared for a night of croup (see Chapter Twelve). Sometimes the first sign of impending croup is hoarseness. It may not be the voice box itself that is swollen, but the area right below the voice box (where croup hits) becomes swollen, creating some hoarseness. This may come before the classic barky croup cough that parents of croupy kids know all too well. If you hear some hoarseness in your child who has had croup, prepare in advance, and you may even thwart a bad croup episode. Get the humidifier going, and check with your pediatrician if it is ok to give a dose of steroids (if you have them at home), or ask her to call some in to your local pharmacy. I wouldn't recommend this if your child hasn't had croup in the past, but if she has, and if steroids have worked, treating earlier rather than later (earlier in the croup episode, as well as earlier in the evening!) may nip it in the bud, or at least minimize the severity of the episode.

THE BIG PICTURE

Hoarseness in toddlers and preschoolers is very common. As the voice box grows, the delicate vocal cords become longer than those of an infant, making them stronger, yet more susceptible to overuse injury. Infant vocal cords are very short, and very slippery, which is one of the reasons why infants are rarely hoarse, even if they cry for most of their waking hours. Toddlers are spirited by nature, and will use their efforts without bounds. This includes the use of their voices. They will yell louder than anyone in order to be heard, shriek with glee, or cry with vigor. Some will do this daily, and become hoarse. If it is temporary, no evaluation or treatment is needed, except maybe some behavior modification. But if they have chronic hoarseness for more than four weeks (either hoarseness that appears daily, does not change throughout the day, or progresses to the point of worsening hoarseness, loss of voice, or even breathing difficulty), a medical evaluation is warranted. Have your pediatrician take a look first, but an ear, nose, and throat specialist will need to take a look at the vocal cords directly to see what's going on. Most causes of hoarseness in children can be treated with some lifestyle changes (learning to be quiet, for starters), but rare disorders need more intensive medical treatments.

DON'T WORRY

If your chatty child is occasionally hoarse, there is little to worry about. Many kids use their voices in unusual ways, but more likely they are just using it in loud ways. As long as he is not hoarse most of the time, there is likely just some transient swelling of the vocal cords on especially 'loud' days. Some gentle reminders about volume control will eventually sink in. Likely, these will be adhered to at school more so than at home. Gently remind older children and adults about volume control, as it's usually not your loud toddler who is the only culprit.

WORRY

If your child has hoarseness that progresses to the point where she either loses her voice completely, has a very raspy/breathy voice that is down to a whisper, or has any signs of breathing trouble at all, she should have a medical evaluation. If your child was diagnosed with asthma but is hoarse, she needs to see an ear, nose, and throat specialist. Asthma does not cause hoarseness. Hoarseness can be associated with wheezing, but asthma is a disease of the lower airways, not the voice box. If your child is eating or playing with something in his mouth and suddenly chokes and becomes hoarse, the object (food or otherwise) may be on or around the voice box. If he can talk, have him try to cough it out. If he cannot talk, use the Heimlich maneuver to try to extract the object. Go to the emergency room or call 911 if he is having any trouble breathing, or if the hoarseness is getting worse.

TO-DO LIST: HOARSENESS IN TODDLERS AND PRESCHOOLERS: SHHHHHHH!

1. Many children have transient hoarseness. If yours does, try to track when it comes and goes. If you hear it at the end of each day, work on strategies to modulate volume at home and at school — this goes for the whole family.

2. If your child is hoarse for more than one month, even if it goes away each morning, an ear, nose, and throat specialist should check for 'screamer's nodules' or other growths.

3. Voice therapy is a great source for educating you, your child, and family members about volume control.

4. If your child has progressive hoarseness, loss of voice for more than three months, loss of voice to a whisper, or any breathing trouble stemming from hoarseness, seek medical attention from your pediatrician, who can refer you to a specialist.

5. If your child has had croup, and sounds hoarse, it may be the early stages of croup. Be prepared.

6. If your child develops sudden hoarseness after choking on food or a toy, or any foreign object, it is possible that the object is lodged on or around the voice box. Do not try the Heimlich maneuver if your child can speak, but encourage him to cough it out. If he is having any breathing trouble, bring him to an emergency room or call 911.

Sources for Hoarseness in Toddlers:
www.rrpf.org
www.pediatric-ent.com/learning/problems/vocalcord

Chapter Nineteen

Wheezing and Coughing: When is it Asthma?

Wheezing during early childhood, especially when associated with a cold or cough, is often termed 'Reactive Airway Disease' (RAD) or 'infant asthma', and it may eventually go away. However, young children (even those under three years of age) with chronic or relapsing symptoms such as wheezing and coughing may have early signs of asthma. Asthma is one of the most common causes of hospitalization in children, and accounts for one third of emergency room visits in children. It is also the fourth most common reason for a child to visit the pediatrician, and it is the most common chronic illness in children. More than nine million children in the United States are asthmatic, and this number continues to rise. Nobody has the answer as to why asthma has become more and more common, but one possible explanation is because of rising levels of pollution. While, overall air quality in the U.S. has improved, studies have shown that if a child lives near a highly congested traffic area, such as a freeway, they are at increased risk of developing asthma. Another possible reason is the increase in greenhouse gases, which may in turn, lead to increase in pollen levels. High pollen levels may trigger asthma-type symptoms in children with environmental allergies, and 70% of asthmatics have environmental allergies. Another possible reason for the rise in asthma prevalence is that children are being more sequestered in their early years, which may make their immune system more fragile when they eventually come into contact with other children. In fact, a recent study showed that daycare attendance in early toddlerhood actually lowered a child's chances of developing asthma.

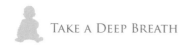

Since asthma is a type of 'reactive airway disease', asthma symptoms are usually brought on by some type of irritant, such as allergens, tobacco smoke, air pollution, or a respiratory illness such as cold, sinus infection, or bronchitis. Children with asthma require very close medical attention, both at home and outside the home. As your child gets older, he will be able to take on more responsibility in recognizing and treating his symptoms.

Other possible causes of wheezing may include rare disorders of the windpipe (**trachea**), rare chronic lung disorders such as **cystic fibrosis**, or food-choking episodes.

My two-year-old coughs for weeks at a time after each cold that he gets. He runs and plays normally, but coughs all day and all night. Is this asthma?

Most commonly when there is residual coughing, especially with running around, or at night, following a respiratory illness, a form of 'reactive airway disease' is the cause. This is seen specifically in the setting of an otherwise well child, who has no fevers, irritability, lethargy, or loss of appetite. Your child will seem 'fine', but coughs regularly. The cough may be dry, hacking, or slightly 'moist' and there will most likely be no actual 'wheezing'. While your pediatrician may be able to hear wheezing with a stethoscope, you will not actually hear a wheeze in your child's breathing. Your child's lower airways (bronchi and lungs) are 'reacting' to residual swelling or mucus from the respiratory illness, thus the term 'reactive' airway disease – the airways are literally 'reacting'.

When coughing ('reacting') persists following a respiratory infection, your pediatrician may want to give your child a trial of breathing treatments. These breathing treatments act to (1) reduce the swelling in the airways, allowing the mucus to clear and (2) open up the airways that have become narrowed from swelling and mucus. A medication called **budesonide (Pulmicort®)** is an inhaled steroid, which acts to reduce swelling and inflammation in the airways (bronchi and lungs). A second medication called **levalbuterol (Xopenex®)** acts as a **bronchodilator**, opening up the narrowed bronchi in the lungs. These medications can be used either separately or together, depending on what your doctor recommends. Their function is to reduce the chronic coughing caused by airway irritation.

You may hear your doctor use the term 'cough-variant asthma' if coughing is the only symptom, in the absence of wheezing. Some children only need to use these breathing medications during and immediately following respiratory illnesses. Some need to use them all the time, depending on how chronic their coughing becomes. Some will only need to use them during the respiratory illness seasons (usually Fall and Winter). Yet another group will use one of the medications (usually budesonide) all of the time, and levalbuterol and budesonide when an illness flares up. A third medication sometimes recommended to reduce coughing and wheezing is **ipratropium bromide (Atrovent®)**. This medication is a bronchodilator, similar in action to albuterol. It does not work immediately during an acute flare, but acts to prevent wheezing by relaxing and opening the air passages. It can be used in children who are five years and older.

True 'asthma' itself is very difficult to diagnose in young children, because it requires cooperation for breathing assessments. These breathing assessments (**pulmonary function tests**) require that the child breathes as hard as he can into a tube. The strength of his breath will be recorded on a machine, which will determine whether there is a lung problem or not, and how to treat it. A trial of long-term 'control' therapy such as inhaled steroids is recommended for younger children. This medication, when used on a regular basis can, block symptoms such as coughing and wheezing during and after respiratory illnesses.

Young children who have had four or more episodes of wheezing during one year, two episodes in six months, or more than two days per week of symptoms in a four-week period, are candidates for long-term therapies. Most doctors recommend starting with inhaled steroids, such as budesonide. If therapy does not show reduction in symptoms within 4–6 weeks, your doctor may consider other therapies or diagnoses. If therapy is showing improvement, then your doctor may attempt to find the lowest dosage and frequency of the medications that can control your child's symptoms.

My son's allergist recommended that my four-year-old should begin taking a medication called montelukast for his wheezing and coughing. Is he too young for this? How does this medication work?

This medication, commonly known as Singulair®, is safe for children as young as one-year-old, according to the FDA. It can be given as chewable tablets or as dissolvable granules. It acts by blocking the receptors involved in the very early stages of an allergic response, even before your child is exposed to a particular allergen. In that sense, it can be used as a preventative medication in allergic children, if used

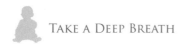

on a regular basis. If your child's coughing and wheezing are related to allergies, this medication prevents the allergic trigger.

What if my child is still having coughing and wheezing, despite being on inhaled steroids and bronchodilators?

For more severe forms of reactive airway disease or asthma, the frequency of medication administration may need to be adjusted based on your child's symptoms. For these severe cases, children may need these inhaled medications four times per day. Rarely, when symptoms become worse, children may need a short course of oral steroids (**prednisone**) to help reduce the airway swelling.

My 20-month-old started having a cough a few weeks ago.
She doesn't seem sick, but she coughs both day and night, on and off.
A week before she started coughing, she slept at my parents' house.
I noticed that they fed her some pistachios, which she seemed to love.

While all may be well and good, it is possible that one of those tasty nuts is sitting in your child's lower windpipe. Even if she didn't have a choking episode, little fragments may have found their way down 'the wrong pipe'. Telltale signs of a 'silent' food choking event are 'new-onset' cough after a new food was eaten, leading to wheezing. An astute pediatrician will recognize that your child has 'asthma on one side', since the wheezing will only occur on the side where the food fragments lie. If a chest X-ray is done, there may be asymmetric air patterns comparing one lung to the other (radiologists refer to this classic sign of blockage as 'air trapping'). A wise allergist once sent me such a patient (in his case it was peanuts), who had been diagnosed with asthma, allergies, bronchitis, you name it, for over three months. He told me 'Nina, there's something down there — maybe a nut. This kid only wheezes on his right side!'. Lo and behold, by the time I looked, it was peanut butter down there. Butter got removed, asthma got cured.

My three-year-old has a deep, wet cough that hasn't gotten any better with nebulizers, antibiotics, allergy medications, or steroids. My doctor wants her to be tested for cystic fibrosis. What is this?

Cystic fibrosis is a chronic inflammatory disorder of several organ systems, most notably of the lungs, sinuses, and gastrointestinal (digestive) system. Symptoms can be as mild as an occasional sinus infection, to severe life-threatening lung and breathing disease. The disorder leads to thick mucus build-up in the respiratory system (lungs and sinuses), leading to bronchitis, sinusitis, and pneumonia. Severe cases are usually diagnosed soon after birth, but very mild cases may go undiagnosed until adulthood. In general, children are diagnosed before the age of three years, by either having had lung infections or digestive issues. These children will have frequent bronchitis, which may lead to pneumonias. The classic test for cystic fibrosis is called a **sweat chloride test**. This is a painless test, performed by gathering a small amount of sweat from the skin. An abnormal amount of chloride (one of the chemicals in salt – sodium chloride) indicates likelihood of cystic fibrosis. Nowadays, there are many genetic tests that can be performed (and several genes have been identified) for presence of cystic fibrosis. Parents can also be screened for having the gene for cystic fibrosis before or during pregnancy. Both parents need to carry the same gene for cystic fibrosis in order for them to have a 50% chance of having a child with the disease.

If your child is diagnosed with cystic fibrosis, while it is a challenging disease, you should know that the treatments have become much more successful over the last ten to twenty years. Over 30,000 people in the United States alone have cystic fibrosis, and the quality of life and life expectancy have grown exponentially since the early years of treatment. Specialized care from multiple disciplines is needed (pediatrics, pulmonology, otolaryngology, gastroenterology, allergy/immunology), but many large medical facilities have outstanding care centers to treat both children and adults with this disease.

My 15-month-old has this strange, brassy cough. He has had it for months, but he doesn't seem sick at all. It doesn't slow him down, except when he needs to stop and cough.

If any lung issue has been ruled out, it may be that your child's funny cough may be coming from his windpipe. Very rarely, children are born with floppy areas in the windpipe. The strength and integrity of the windpipe should be similar to that of a bicycle tire, but occasionally it can be similar to that of the tire's inner tube. If the windpipe is more like an inner tube, the front and back walls of the windpipe will hit up against each other when your child coughs, creating a 'brassy' or 'honking' sound. The technical term for this is **tracheomalacia** (floppy trachea). Tracheomalacia

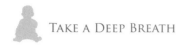

can be due to an integral floppiness of the trachea itself, or it can be caused by something pushing up against it (a blood vessel, or the way the heart lies in the chest) causing a floppy area. Diagnosis is made by an ear, nose, and throat doctor or a pulmonary doctor who can look down the windpipe with a tiny camera. Your child will have to be asleep for this procedure, for about 15 to 20 minutes. In addition (or alternatively), a specialized X-ray (**computed tomography, or CT Scan**) or **Magnetic Resonance Imaging** (MRI) scan of the area can identify the site of floppiness, and whether or not anything from the surrounding structures is causing the floppiness. Most children with tracheomalacia eventually grow out of it, as the windpipe gains some strength. Very VERY rarely, children need surgery to either repair the weakness or lift away the structure causing the floppiness.

My two-and-a-half-year-old seems to cough a lot after drinking milk. My doctor recommended cutting out dairy from his diet. Is he allergic to dairy?

In general, dairy foods tend to have some effect on almost everyone: they increase the acid secretion in the stomach, and they tend to thicken the mucus that is already there. The increase in release of stomach acid can sometimes contribute to **gastroesophageal reflux**, whereby microscopic food and/or acid particles come up the esophagus, to the back of the throat. This may cause irritation and coughing. The association with dairy products and thickened mucus can also lead to coughing. Many patients tell me that cutting out dairy helps their child's symptoms. My response is that it sounds great, but make sure that your child's nutrition is not being compromised, and perhaps try different types of dairy products at different times of the day to see if it's a blanket 'no dairy' regimen. A true dairy *allergy* is something that has to be assessed by *allergy* testing. A dairy allergy is usually associated with serious reactions, anywhere from hives on the skin, to vomiting, diarrhea, bloody diarrhea, or even breathing problems. Difficulty in breathing in response to a food or environmental allergen is called **anaphylaxis**. Any breathing problem related to an exposure of any kind requires emergency treatment. If your child experiences this for the first time, call 911. If your child has a known history of a severe food allergy, you will most likely have something called an **Epi-pen** (a single-dose injectable epinephrine treatment to be given in such an emergency).

Before receiving one of these, your doctor's office will give you specific instructions on how and when to do this.

Dairy *intolerance* is something completely different, and symptoms are usually exclusively digestive (bloating, gas cramps, diarrhea). This reaction is usually due to an insufficient amount of a particular **enzyme** (lactase), which is responsible for breaking down one of the sugars in dairy products (lactose). There are many lactose-free dairy products that can be substituted, without having to cut out dairy altogether. Many parents note that dairy-induced coughing (when not truly allergy-based) is transient, and in most children, dairy can be slowly re-introduced over time. A common reason that dairy products 'cause' coughing is that they are given in the bed or crib, or given right before naptime or bedtime. If your child is going to have any coughing from dairy products, that's the time they'll do it.

Cutting out milk at bedtime (certainly in the bed) may cut down coughing. However, it will certainly not cut down any crying. Toddlers are quite routinized, and even changing the color of the bottle or sippy cup may be traumatic, let alone changing its contents (water is fine, any time). This battle, unfortunately, goes back to sleep training, but on a more difficult level. Compromise may work, and more importantly, will preserve what little sanity you may have with a cranky toddler. You can of course try explaining the change to him: 'Bottle at bedtime, but we'll sit and read a story while you have it. Then to bed like a big boy'. 'Bottle in your bed, but water in the bottle'. Or, you can gradually (ever so gradually – kids are smarter than we think), dilute the milk each night until it's water. They'll figure it out of course, but hopefully by that time you'll be halfway there.

My three-year-old seems to cough and wheeze in the Spring months. Is she too young to see an allergist?

No. She is not too young. While allergies (environmental, such as dust, pollen, and animal hair) are more notable in older children, children as young as two years old can show signs of allergies. Many of these children have family members with allergies, or they may have had skin sensitivities such as eczema as infants. They may or may not have stuffy noses, but may have signs of asthma-like breathing issues such as coughing and wheezing. If the trigger of such difficulties is a particular allergen or multiple allergens, treatment, which may include either removing the source if

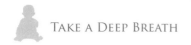

possible and/or **anti-histamine** medications, is an option for toddlers as well as older children.

My four-year-old has asthma. My neighbor in the apartment next to ours smokes. Moving is not an option, nor is convincing my neighbor to quit smoking. Will an air purifier help?

HEPA (high-efficiency, particle-arresting) air purifiers have been shown to reduce the number of emergency visits for asthmatic patients, even when children are exposed to second-hand smoke. However, while they reduce the amount of particle contaminants, they do not reduce the amount of gas toxins in tobacco smoke. Suffice it to say that there is no 'safe' level of second hand smoke exposure for children, especially for those with breathing issues.

My five-year-old used to use a nebulizer, but now I think he's ready for an inhaler. What's the difference, and how do I know if he's ready to switch over?

The method of medication administration is really up to you and your child. All methods have similar benefits, assuming they are administered correctly. Most younger children do better with a nebulizer, which provides a visible mist from a machine. No breath coordination is needed, and a parent, caregiver, or child can hold the mask. Inhalers, on the other hand, especially for older kids, have several advantages: They are more portable, and do not require a power source such as a battery or outlet needed for a nebulizer machine. They deliver the medication much more quickly than a nebulizer. Unlike the gradual release of medicated steam from a nebulizer, an inhaler gives all of the medication in one or two inhaled puffs. A 'metered dose inhaler' (MDI) requires some coordination, as your child must be able to activate the device and inhale quickly, all at the same time. Most kids over five or six can master this. Many doctors, however, will include a 'spacer' with an inhaler. You or your child can fill the spacer with the set amount of medicine, and then your child can use the inhaler. The spacer provides the appropriate dose of medication between the medication source and the inhaler, enabling him to receive the correct amount without the need to coordinate the activation of the inhaler's pump with his breathing.

THE BIG PICTURE

Infants and young children should not wheeze during or after a cold. If they do, they need to be evaluated by their doctor. Chronic coughing or wheezing after recovery from an illness may be a sign of 'infant asthma' or 'reactive airway disease'. While these children are a bit more likely than others to go on to develop true asthma, it is certainly not always the case. There are wide ranges of wheezing and coughing, ranging from those that have it only when sick, those who have it only during and after illnesses, those who have it only during the cold and flu season, to those who have it all the time. Many safe medications exist to manage these symptoms, and the exact regimen can be tailored to your child's needs. Other causes of wheezing in this age group are less common, although not less significant. Rare lung and windpipe disorders may need to be investigated, or delving into a history of a food choking episode may be revealed. In any event, wheezing needs to be heard by your doctor.

DON'T WORRY

If your child has coughing and/or wheezing following colds, this is very likely something that can be managed safely by your pediatrician. Many medication options exist, both as nebulizers (breathing treatments) and oral medications. Your primary pediatrician may or may not ask you to see an allergist (if allergies seem to be the source) or a pulmonary (lung) specialist if your child's symptoms are a bit tricky to manage. Many kids with wheezing issues as toddlers grow out of these issues as their air passages and immune systems mature. Use of nebulizers for your child does not necessarily mean a lifetime of breathing treatments. And if that is her destiny, you will be amazed at how quickly it becomes incorporated into her life, without slowing her down.

WORRY

Sudden onset wheezing or coughing is always worrisome. It implies that there is a sudden change, or blockage in the air passages. Did your child choke on something? Did you miss a treatment this afternoon? Is he sicker than you think (for instance did he spike a high fever, possibly indicating bronchitis or pneumonia?). Any sudden change in breathing means that your child needs medical attention. Go to the emergency room or call 911. Don't worry alone!

TO-DO LIST: WHEEZING AND COUGHING: WHEN IS IT ASTHMA?

1. If you think your child's cough is lasting too long following a cold, have it checked out. You may notice that she coughs throughout the whole day, or you may notice that her cough is worse at night. Either way, kids should stop coughing within a few days of a cold's resolution. Have her doctor check her if it doesn't go away.

2. Wheezing cannot always be heard without a stethoscope. Don't go out and buy one yourself. Let your pediatrician use his. He uses his ears, as well as his training and experience, to make an assessment.

3. If you CAN hear your child wheezing, then she is most likely having some serious breathing difficulties. If she is not already receiving medical therapy, she needs to see a doctor.

4. The importance of milk is underrated, especially in kids. Be sure you really think that milk is the culprit before removing it from your child's diet. If it does seem to cause problems such as coughing, consider gradually introducing other forms of dairy back into his diet over time, especially in the first half of the day.

5. If your child starts wheezing or coughing suddenly, seek medical attention right away.

6. Don't smoke.

7. If you live in a building with smokers, consider purchasing an air purifier. Your child may be getting more tobacco exposure than you think.

Sources for Wheezing and Coughing:
www.nhlbi.nih.gov/guidelines/asthma (accessed 1/18/11)
www.pediatrics.org
www.yourlunghealth.org/medication/desc/ipratropium
www.kidshealth.org/parent/medical/asthma/inhaler_nebulizer
www.cdc.gov.mmwr
www.cff.org
www.webmd.com/asthma/guide/diagnosing-asthma
www.webmd.com/asthma/guide/asthma-treatments
Pediatrics 2011;127:93–101

Chapter Twenty

Respiratory Illnesses in Toddlers and Preschoolers: Yuck!

The toddler and preschool years are really the beginning of what medical specialists gleefully term 'the kiddy krud years'. While toddlers are hearty young beings, they have immature **immune systems** and immature airway structures, often making it hard for them to combat respiratory illnesses. They are also socially and emotionally immature, and hand washing is usually not their first, second or, third priority on their to-do list. However, they are not too young to start understanding that hand washing is part of their many routines, even if they think it's just for fun. And it does make a difference in minimizing rapid spread of both common and uncommon diseases. Kids should be taught that hand washing includes soap AND water (or hand sanitizer if there is no sink available), and that it should last for as long as it takes for them to sing 'happy birthday', 'twinkle twinkle, little star', or the 'abc song'. The hand washer gets to choose the song.

During these years, you will be introduced to illnesses of which you have never heard, but soon phrases such as **'coxsackie virus'**, **'hand–foot–and–mouth disease'** and **'Fifth disease'** will be rolling off your tongue from the playground to the dinner table. This chapter will give you the down and dirty (and I mean *dirty*) of these 'yuck' illnesses of childhood.

My two-year-old was sent home from daycare because she was running a fever. She seemed fine this morning, but had a little runny nose. Is this just a cold?

In all likelihood, it is just a cold. But fever of any kind is reason enough to send your child home, both for her protection and for the protection of the kids and caretakers

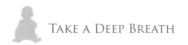

around her. When you get her home (after you've frantically cancelled your work meeting and afternoon appointments), check her temperature yourself, and see how she seems overall. Is she playful? Cranky? Lethargic? Make sure you ask your daycare provider if any medication such as **ibuprofen** or **acetominophen** was given, and, if so, how much and at what time. Also, ask if there has been 'something going around' (99% of the time the answer will be 'yes'), but if there is any specific illness that week, it may give you a clue as to what you're in for.

Fevers and fever medicine need to be tracked very carefully. I suggest you break out a clean pad of paper and keep track of time, temperature, and medicine given. You will be surprised how quickly the hours will blend into each other when you have a sick child. Ibuprofen OR acetominophen can be given up to every three hours to keep a fever down. Push fluids as much as you can, and, for high fevers, you can give your child a warm bath (do not give a cold bath or an ice bath — these were done when I was a kid, but can cause chills or even seizures, and won't bring down a fever any faster than a warm bath). You can place cool wet washcloths on your child's head or forehead, but keep the rest of her body covered so she does not get chills. If the fever doesn't break with these measures, then it's time to call the doctor. There are so many causes of a fever, so, especially if it's not breaking, see what your doctor recommends. Common colds can cause a fever, but the fever is usually mild (under 101°F), and comes down with fever-reducing medications such as acetominophen or ibuprofen. Fevers from a flu, an ear infection, gastro-intestinal illnesses, and severe bacterial or viral infections are not as easy to control.

If it turns out to be just a cold, keep your child at home until she is fever-free for at least one day (without needing fever medication). This will ensure that she is well enough to return, is not contagious, and will not be sent home yet again for an incompletely resolved illness.

My three-year-old had a cold two days ago. Today she woke up with bright red cheeks and a funny rash on her body. What's going on?

Does it look like someone slapped her cheeks? Does the rest of the rash look a bit like pink lace? It may be something called **Fifth Disease**. The name is derived because it is the fifth of the classic illnesses that cause rashes in children (measles, rubella, scarlet fever, and an unnamed 'fourth' disease are the others). This is a surprisingly common illness seen in daycares, preschools, and even elementary schools. It classically begins as what seems like a very mild cold (stuffy or runny nose, mild fever, cough), which goes away. After the cold symptoms subside, a rash breaks out. It may be only on the cheeks, (which will look bright red as if they were slapped), or it may also involve the torso, arms and legs (these areas will have a fine, lacy, pink appearance). The rash is usually smooth to touch and does not itch. Most kids have the rash for a few days, with minimal or no symptoms. Fifth disease is very contagious (it is caused by a virus called **parvovirus B19**), but the contagious period is during the alleged 'cold', not during the rash (so, yes, you can send your child to daycare with a Fifth disease rash — assuming she is not in pain and not having a fever). Rarely children will also have fever and joint pain with the rash, which can be treated with ibuprofen, and very rarely, steroids. Because it is so contagious, and because the presence of Fifth disease is not known at the time of contagion, it tends to occur in outbreaks. Most adults have antibodies to the disease (meaning they are immune to it, having had some mild exposure, or the disease itself, at some point in childhood), but occasionally adults can develop Fifth disease along with their children. As in most instances when an adult contracts a childhood illness, the symptoms are worse — a worse rash, a higher fever, and more joint pain. One of the many sacrifices of parenthood! The good news is that you can only get Fifth Disease once.

My 18-month-old was up all night screaming. He had a fever this morning, so I took him to the doctor. My doctor showed me the horrible looking sores at the back of his throat. Where did he get this?
He could have gotten this anywhere — daycare, friends, the park, toddler group, the mall, a sibling, or a neighbor. Horrible looking ulcers (and they are as painful as they look) are caused by a virus called **coxsackie virus**. This is a very common, and very contagious virus seen in toddlers and preschoolers. The virus can also affect the palms and soles, with similar ulcers or blisters on these surfaces. Because of these three common sites, the illness is cleverly called **hand–foot–and–mouth disease**. Anyone who's gone through this with their young one can attest to the fact that it is, indeed, truly awful — mainly because the sores are quite painful, and there is no magic (or real) cure. Because this disease is caused by a virus, no antibiotics will get rid of

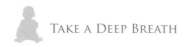

the illness. Treatment involves simply treating the symptoms with pain medicine (ibuprofen or acetaminophen), and time. Most kids have the painful sores only for a few days, but some can have them for up to a week.

Some patients feel some relief if their doctor prescribes an oral solution called 'one to one to one', which consists of equal parts of Benadryl®, Kaopectate®, and lidocaine. A prescription is needed for this, and it can be prepared by a pharmacist. For young children (18 months in this scenario), it can be applied with an unused paintbrush or cotton ball to the roof of the mouth. Older children can use it as a 'swish and spit', but it shouldn't be swallowed. Some pain relief, especially inside the mouth, is very important, especially in small children, because they must continue to eat (or at least drink) so as not to get dehydrated. This is yet another disease that usually occurs in 'outbreaks'. Unlike Fifth disease, coxsackie virus infections can occur more that once.

My four-year-old has what seems like pink eye, but is also quite sick, with high fever, sore throat, and a sore neck. What can this be?

Another very contagious virus (are you getting the theme of this chapter yet?) is **adenovirus**. This is a very common virus, similar to the cold viruses, but it usually causes worse symptoms. It can affect the eyes, leading to redness, sticky drainage, and itching, accompanied by fever, fatigue, sore throat, and swollen **lymph nodes** ('glands') in the neck. It spreads very quickly from person to person, and thus is also seen in outbreaks. Symptoms can be mild (low grade fever, mild sore throat) to severe (high fevers, severe throat pain, severe neck pain, severe redness of the eyes, and even diarrhea). It usually lasts anywhere from three to ten days, and treatment, as for most of the viruses, involves treating the symptoms.

My 15-month-old received the flu vaccine (including H1N1), but my doctor told me that he has the flu. How did this happen?

The American Academy of Pediatrics recommends that all children over the age of six months receive the flu vaccine. In the first year that she receives immunization she will need two separate vaccinations, at least one month apart, in order to develop immunity for that flu season. While the flu vaccine covers most strains of the flu virus (including H1N1), there are some strains that are not covered, and thousands of vaccinated people each year nonetheless suffer from a full-on case of the flu. It is not possible to create a flu vaccine that prevents all strains of the flu. New flu strains are continually being formed, by spontaneous mutations of viruses. As with other respiratory viruses, all flu viruses are very contagious. Unfortunately, having been vaccinated does not mean that the illness will be milder, and this disease, especially in young children, needs to be taken seriously. Fever during the flu tends to run very high (in the 103–105°F range), and you will need to monitor temperature closely. Take notes on time of the fever, medication given, and whether the fever broke with the medication. Babies and toddlers are at high risk for dehydration during the flu: the combination of the high fever, lethargy, and disinterest in food or drink makes this situation especially worrisome. In these situations, don't worry about food or milk. Just focus on fluids. Water is good, but something with some **electrolytes** such as Pedialyte® or even diluted sport drinks (those without caffeine) are an even better option. If your child has a dry diaper for more than twelve hours in this setting, give your doctor a call. He may want you to either come in for a check, or he may even ask you to go to an emergency room. If a child is dehydrated, he often feels nauseated, making it even less enticing for him to eat or drink. He may even vomit from dehydration, making him even more dehydrated. It then becomes a vicious cycle. In an emergency room, your child may receive some intravenous fluids for hydration. Being hydrated will make him feel better, and perhaps even interested in drinking something. Doctors may also want to do some blood tests for signs of a bacterial infection, to assess the degree of dehydration, and to look for any signs of electrolyte imbalance. He may also perform a chest X-ray. Thousands of children each year develop pneumonia as a complication from the flu, and an X-ray will determine whether or not your child's lungs are free of infection.

Medications such as **Tamiflu®** and **Relenza®** have been recommended to reduce the duration of the illness associated with the flu, and can be given to children over 12 months old. While these medications do not cure the flu, they have been shown to reduce the duration of the illness by one to two days. There are preparations that are safe for infants and toddlers, and may be prepared in liquid form — just check with your pediatrician for dosing and potential side effects. These can only be given by prescription.

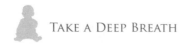
My 18-month old had a cold with a fever three days ago. She woke up this morning with a red/pink rash on her chest and stomach. Later today the rash spread to her arms and legs. She's not sick anymore, and the rash doesn't seem to bother her, but it looks really awful. Is she contagious?

Occasionally after a respiratory illness, your child may break out in a rash covering most of her body. This may be an entity termed **roseola (exanthem subitum, or Sixth Disease)**. This awful looking rash is actually quite benign. The contagious time was during the respiratory illness itself, so once the rash breaks out, your child is no longer contagious. The rash can last from three to seven days, and is commonly seen in toddlers and even in infants as young as six months old. No treatment is necessary. It will go away on its own. If you are not sure that your child's rash is caused by roseola, have your doctor take a look.

My five-year-old has a sore throat, fever, and stomach ache. My doctor wants her to come to the office for a Strep test. If she has Strep throat, will she need her tonsils to be taken out?

There are many reasons for a sore throat, and most of them are that your child has a virus. But Strep throat is caused by a type of bacteria (**Streptococcus**) that usually infects the tonsils. The tonsils (one on each side of the back of the throat) are lymph nodes that both fight infection as well as become infected. Bacteria and viruses like to grow in the tonsil tissue, and can cause swelling, redness, pain, and even white or yellow spots on the tonsils. Your doctor can take a swab of your child's throat, on or near the tonsils. All kids hate this — it makes them gag when they are already down and out, but it's important. A rapid strep test can be performed in most pediatricians' offices, and it is a 'quick look' test for strep. You will have the results of 'positive' or 'negative' in less than five minutes. If the rapid strep test is positive, your child will be given a prescription for antibiotics, usually in the penicillin family, or if your child is allergic to penicillin, another antibiotic which also kills the strep bacteria. If the rapid strep test is negative, the sample will be sent for a culture, and the results usually take 24 to 48 hours. If the culture is negative, then the sore throat is viral, and no antibiotics are needed. If the culture is positive, your child will need antibiotics. A rare, although not unheard of, complication of strep throat is **scarlet fever**.

This can occur even if your child is receiving antibiotics, and is associated with a rash, usually all over the body, with tiny red, raised bumps. There is usually a high fever as well, lasting several days to a week. **Rheumatic fever** was a complication of strep seen in the era before penicillin, and involved a strep infection of the heart valves, eventually leading to lifelong heart problems.

If your child has one (or even a few) episodes of strep throat (strep tonsillitis), she does not necessarily need to have her tonsils removed, especially if she is not having symptoms related to breathing problems such as snoring, sleep apnea, or difficulty breathing during sleep. The American Academy of Otolaryngology guidelines for tonsil removal based on recurrent throat infections states that seven infections in one year, five infections per year for two years, or three infections per year for at least three years, are indications to consider tonsillectomy. So, for now, she can keep her tonsils. But make sure she takes her full course of antibiotics, as directed and on schedule.

Which vaccines are recommended after the first year?

Most of the vaccines and/or boosters are given in your child's first year. However, some are given at either the 12- or the 15-month visit, so make sure you stay on track with your pediatrician visits. At your child's 12-month visit, your doctor will let you know whether or not your child needs to return for more immunizations at 15 months. After that, immunizations become fewer at each visit, and less frequent, except for the flu shot — or flumist — which should be given annually to you, your child, older siblings, and caregivers.

12–15 months:
- ❖ Hemophilus influenzae (Hib)
- ❖ Pneumococcal vaccine (PCV)
- ❖ Measles, Mumps, Rubella (MMR)
- ❖ Varicella ('chicken pox vaccine')
- ❖ Hepatitis A (two doses)

15–18 months
- ❖ Diphtheria, Tetanus, Pertussis (DTaP)

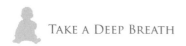

4–6 years

❖ Diphtheria, Tetanus, Pertussis (DTaP)
❖ Inactivated Poliovirus Vaccine (IPV)
❖ Measles, Mumps, Rubella (MMR) (blood levels of immunity to MMR may be drawn, and if immunity to these viruses is present, booster may be withheld)
❖ Varicella

THE BIG PICTURE

The toddler and preschool years are times to keep your (locked) medicine chest stocked with fever medications, nasal saline, and thermometers. Have a few of these — they get misplaced remarkably easily. Expect many respiratory illnesses during this time. Kids get an average of ten colds per year, which is nearly one per month. This will make it seem as if they are 'always sick'. This is not too far from the truth, and if you have more than one child, you may at times, feel like you're running a full-time infirmary, with a very fast revolving door. Most of these illnesses are simple colds, usually seen as a runny and/or stuffy nose, mild 'wet' cough, possibly a low-grade fever (up to 100°F), and perhaps some irritability. When high fevers and weird rashes come into play, other possible causes need to be explored. Many cold viruses (and flu viruses) will lead to high fever, but if the fever is not controlled with acetominophen and/or ibuprofen, your pediatrician needs a call. Depending on other symptoms, such as a bad cough, not eating or drinking, or lethargy, she may want to examine your child in the office. Treatment for viral infections is 'supportive' (meaning, treat the symptoms), but bacterial infections will require antibiotics.

DON'T WORRY

If your child has what seems to you to be frequent colds, he is probably in good company with his friends. Toddlers are constantly exploring the world boundlessly, have little or no etiquette about personal space and possessions, and certainly no concerns regarding cleanliness. Daycare and preschools are laden with toys, floor time, inadvertently shared snacks, shared tissues, and shared illnesses. Even the best of caregivers and teachers can't always keep up with the mayhem. As long as your child recovers within three to five days from most colds, frequency (up to one per month, sometimes two in the fall and winter months) is within the norm. If your child develops a fever, he should receive medication to bring the fever down (acetaminophen or ibuprofen), and the fever should come down within 30 to 60 minutes of taking the medication. If your child is able to drink, sleep comfortably, and has wet diapers (or is peeing in the potty), there is little to worry about. If your child develops a rash at any point during or after a respiratory illness, do not panic. Most rashes occur after an illness, and are not contagious. Do call your doctor, though. Usually a clear history followed by a clear description of the rash will enable your doctor to determine whether or not your child needs to be seen.

WORRY

If your child has what seem to be 'relentless' colds that seem to never end for months on end, there may be some inciting factor that needs to be addressed. While most sources are not worrisome *per se*, prolonged (greater than two weeks) frequent (more than one per month) colds need to be investigated. Possible reasons for such illnesses may include sinusitis, weak immune system, allergies, enlarged adenoids and/or tonsils, or childhood asthma (reactive airway disease).

If your child has a persistent high fever (greater than 102 or 103°F) that will not come down with fever medication, warm baths, or drinking fluids, call your doctor, especially if your child seems listless or lethargic. It may be a sign of a more serious problem such as pneumonia and/or dehydration.

TO-DO LIST: RESPIRATORY ILLNESSES IN TODDLERS AND PRESCHOOLERS: YUCK!

1. Teach hand washing early — before your child can walk.

2. Teach your child that hand washing involves soap, and the 'abc song'.

3. Expect your child to get colds. Some of these will be mild, but some may be pretty bad.

4. Teach your child to 'cover your cough' and 'cover your sneeze' — coughing and sneezing should be done into the crook of his arm, not into his hand, which will no doubt be in direct contact with another child's hand, snack, shirt, or toy within seconds.

5. Call your pediatrician (or go to an emergency room) if:

    a. Your child refuses to drink for more than six hours (during the daytime).

    b. Your child tries to drink, but keeps throwing up for more than six hours.

    c. Your child has dry diapers (or is not peeing in the potty) for more than twelve hours.

    d. Your child's fever does not go below 101°F with acetaminophen or ibuprofen.

    e. Your child has any breathing trouble.

    f. Your child seems lethargic or especially sleepy.

    g. Your child just 'doesn't seem right'.

6. If your child develops a rash during or soon after an illness, give your doctor a call. Try to describe it as best as possible over the phone ('smooth', 'itchy', 'bumps', 'patchy') as well as its location.

7. Make sure you keep your child on track with his immunization schedule.

8. Make sure your child gets immunized against influenza every year.

9. Most flu shots become available in the late summer/early fall.

10. Make sure you (and all of his caregivers) get a flu shot as well.

Sources for Respiratory Illnesses in Toddlers and Preschoolers:

www.aap.org

www.entnet.org

Clinical practice guideline: Tonsillectomy in Children. Supplement to Otolaryngology — Head Neck Surgery. (Baugh et al.). 144;(1): January 2011.

Chapter Twenty-One
Clear the Air for Your Child

As your child has progressed from the safety of your cocoon to your home to the outside world, his environment becomes less and less in your control. When you were pregnant, you could control what you ate, whether you went to a non-smoking restaurant, and after finally reading those warnings at the gas pump, whether you would avoid pumping gas for your own car — either splurging on full service or asking your spouse or partner to fill your tank. You had some control over your baby's environment — breast or bottle, which type of plastic bottle, which formula, when to choose organic peas, what was the best childcare arrangement, and which park or playground seemed the cleanest and safest. But as your child is introduced to a more independent life as a toddler and preschooler, you will slowly see that many decisions will, sooner than you know or want, be his and not yours. While you still have a somewhat captive audience, this is a great time to start educating your eager-minded tot about his environment — what it can do for him, and what he can (and should) do for it.

What could a child under two possibly learn about the environment?

Certainly one wouldn't expect a child who's just learned to walk to recognize that the ozone layer is in jeopardy. But this is a great age to start learning about 'trash', and where it goes. I never really thought much of trash day until my son was old enough to sit up on his own. He would bounce up and down for joy, wanting to run out to greet the trash truck crew at 6 am every Tuesday. He was not yet a year when his passion for garbage began. It was the perfect time for him to learn about the different color trash trucks and trash bins, and to learn that some trash (recyclables

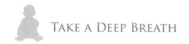
and vegetation) can be used again. By 18 months, we taught him where our recyclable trash goes, as opposed to the trash that is not reusable, so that he could participate in the process. A toddler who is passionate about garbage can also be taught that garbage should be in bins, cans, containers, and garbage trucks. It should not be on the street, at the park, or on his bedroom floor.

When teaching a young toddler about garbage, he must be taught about not putting 'garbage' in his mouth or nose. In this sense of the word, I mean anything but food (or a teething toy/pacifier). While he may not understand that paint on a toy may be toxic, or that today's 'safe' plastic is tomorrow's carcinogen, he must most definitely learn that anything inedible is, indeed, inedible.

How can young children learn that smoking is harmful?

This one really depends on where you live. If you are in an area where there are many smokers, you can let your child know that smoke is 'bad air'. However, with this comment you need to be careful. While as adults we may acknowledge that smokers are hurting themselves, the environment, and those around them, young children can be honest, or worse, judgmental to a fault. If you tell your three-year-old that smoking is stinky, be prepared for her to tell a smoking stranger that they are stinky. Expect some questions — 'Then why do people smoke? ' (or, 'Why does Uncle Bob smoke?', or worse, "Why do you smoke?"). You can tell her that some grown-ups smoke, but they are all really trying to stop, since they know how bad it is for everyone. Thankfully, there is essentially no advertising for cigarettes in public places, on television, or in magazines or movies that children would routinely see.

DO NOT UNDERESTIMATE YOUR TODDLER'S ABILITY TO LEARN GOOD ENVIRONMENTAL HABITS EARLY ON

My four-year-old loves to go to the beach. How can I teach her about air and water pollution if the beach we go to seems pretty clean?

Lucky for you and your daughter that you have a clean beach to enjoy. Unfortunately, this is becoming less and less the norm. If you happen to frequent an unpolluted beach, point out to your daughter how lucky she is to experience it, but that the animals that live at the beach are even luckier. The seagulls do not have to eat styrofoam or plastic, the fish can swim in clean waters, and ocean plant's life can stay vibrant. Show her how plastic and Styrofoam® can look similar to shells and pebbles, and birds can mistakenly eat these inedibles and get really bad tummy aches. You can explain what can happen to the animals and plants if people leave garbage at the beach, if a factory with smokestacks is built at the beach, or if people smoke at the beach. If you live in an area where other beaches (besides your favorite spot) are not so clean, they may be worth a visit, for contrast. If possible, find the most polluted beach in your area, and plan a 'clean up the beach' outing. Bring a trash bag and gardening gloves (or small equivalent for your child) for handling garbage. See if your child can fill the bag. Use a small bag, even the size of a lunch bag, for smaller children. After she's picked up some trash, point out how MUCH she has done by showing what's in the bag, and also point out how MUCH is left on the beach by looking around. The magnitude of the problem will be evident. To bring home the point, con-gratulate your child on how she has made such a BIG difference for this dirty beach (by showing her what's in the bag), but also how BIG a problem pollution is (by looking at the trash along the whole beach and ocean). Many preschools, elementary schools, and other community organizations have more formal 'clean up the beach' (or 'clean up the park', if you are landlocked) days. These are great opportunities for kids as young as two or three to learn about the impact that they can make on cleaning the environment, and also get a sense of the magnitude of the problem. They will very unlikely get the point of pollution, but what they will see is a community of people together, all doing the same thing — cleaning up a big mess. Just as they have 'clean up time' at school and at home, they will get a broader picture of 'clean up time' in their world.

My three-year-old loves to come to the gas station with me, but I don't like him to be exposed to the fumes.

I wouldn't recommend taking your child out of the car to hold the pump, but he can certainly learn that, while for now gasoline is necessary for the majority of car driv-ers, it is indeed stinky. It fills the car's belly and gives it 'energy' to drive, but the

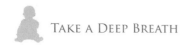

stinky smell goes into the air that we breathe. Too much stinky air is not good for us. This is why we either (1) drive our cars only when necessary, (2) consider a car that doesn't need as much stinky gas, (3) try to carpool with our friends, or (4) use other forms of transportation when we can, such as walking, biking or stroller riding.

My four-year-old wants to help me clean the bathroom. I know this sounds crazy, but he likes to clean the bathtub, his favorite clean-up play place. What cleaning products are safe for him?

It's great that your rugged boy wants to help you clean up his own clean-up place. But keep in mind that cleaning products account for about 10% of toxic exposures in the United States. The worst players are corrosive drain cleaners, oven cleaners, and acidic toilet bowl cleaners.

Years ago, a relatively common childhood injury was accidental lye ingestion (lye is a strong chemical compound called sodium hydroxide, found in many cleaning products). We can thank an otolaryngologist (Dr. Chevalier Jackson), back in the 1920's, for lobbying for passage of the Federal Caustic Poison Act, which required that lye-containing cleaning products contain warning labels. Because cleaning products containing lye were stored in bathroom or kitchen cabinets, and looked like water or juice, kids would accidentally have a drink of this stuff. This would cause an immediate burn to their throat and esophagus, leading to permanent injury and scarring. While we now have the luxury of childproofing and low lye levels in cleaning products, there are still some toxins to avoid around children. Products containing chlorine bleach and ammonia can have toxic fumes. When chorine is combined with ammonia, the two substances react to form chloramine gas, which is also toxic to inhale. When chlorine combines with acid-containing products, chlorine gas, another toxin, is formed.

All cleaning products are labeled, and you should choose those with the 'least toxic' labels. Labels stating 'Poison', 'Flammable', or 'Danger' tend to be the most toxic. Products labeled 'Warning' are moderately hazardous, and products labeled 'Caution' are least hazardous. Other signs of a potentially dangerous product are those stating 'vapors harmful', or 'may cause burns to skin on contact'. Read the product's labels carefully before using the product, especially if there are children in the house. I would be reluctant to have a young child have any direct contact with any cleaning product besides soap and water. Even the most careful child may unknowingly get a bit of product on his hands, and then unknowingly, wipe his eyes, nose, or mouth. Make sure cleaning products, even the 'safe' ones, are in childproofed cabinets, and that these products have safety closures on the bottles. Keep cleaning products stored in their store-bought containers. You don't want your child mistaking a cleaning product for water, soap bubbles, or juice if you store it in a 'child-friendly' bottle. You also want to have access to the name of the product in the event that your child accidentally swallows some. If you think your child accidentally swallowed any part of a cleaning product, call POISON CONTROL at 1-800-222-1222. Do not give your child any water to drink until you speak with someone at poison control and describe exactly what you think the product was. Water can react with some toxic chemicals, forming even more toxic reactions. Do not force your child to vomit. Vomiting the product may result in more damage to the throat, windpipe, and esophagus.

> **THE PHONE NUMBER FOR POISON CONTROL (1-800-222-1222)
> SHOULD BE WRITTEN AND PLACED IN AN EASILY VISIBLE PLACE
> FOR ALL CAREGIVERS TO SEE**

What can I do so my child can model good behavior about caring for his environment?

Kids are excellent mimics, and thankfully, when they are not being obstinate, they are pleasers. "Zero waste" lunches and snacks means no paper or plastic bags — reusable containers only. This is a concept that many daycares, preschools, and elementary schools have instilled. It puts a lot of extra work on parents at the beginning, but it soon becomes second nature. If you continue this 'zero waste' outside of the school by, for example, bringing your own metal coffee container to the coffee shop, bringing your own reusable shopping bags to the market, or using reusable containers for your own lunch or snacks, it will become second nature to your child as well. If he is not accustomed to paper or plastic waste, he will not expect it.

THE BIG PICTURE

As your child becomes more verbal, both in receptive and expressive language, she will become more interactive with the world around her. The toddler and preschool years are the perfect time to begin enabling your child to understand her environment — how it affects her, and how she can affect it. This may be done in 'baby' (or 'toddler' steps). When you are in a beautiful place, explain why it is beautiful: 'Isn't it nice that the trees have so many leaves on them? The birds must love to build nests in them.' 'Look at all of those fish in the pond! Can you guess how many there are?' When you see garbage on the street, at the park, or on the beach, explain how this can be harmful — not just because it looks 'bad' and 'dirty', but because it has a larger impact on their environment as a whole: 'That tree can't get any water to drink because there is so much garbage on the ground around it.' 'The fish don't like swimming in that water because it is too oily and it doesn't taste good to them'. Big concepts are not worth pursuing, but small, tangible concepts such as 'stinky air', 'dirty streets', and 'smoky rooms' may make more sense. Give your child tasks to do, and when dealing with global issues, start from home. Have her help pick which containers to pack snacks or lunch, have her clean her room with you (by age five she should have more independence with this), show her the different color trash bins, and have her help sort recyclables from non-recyclables. The best tool you have that can teach your child about caring for her environment is your own good self. If she sees that you care, both by your actions and by explaining your acts, she will care, too.

DON'T WORRY

When it comes to care for our environment, nobody is perfect. Even the most ecologically-minded adults are not infallible in this area (although they may think they are!). If you drive a gas-guzzler, use plastic or paper grocery bags on occasion, and even buy your daily coffee in a disposable cup, do not feel that you are failing your child, and polluting the world for them and your future grandchildren. But do what you can, within reason, and maybe your child will educate you someday.

WORRY

I've said it before, but since this is heading to the conclusion of this book, I'll say it once again: Do not smoke. It is bad for you, your child, and those around you. Even if you do not smoke in the presence of your child, your clothes carry toxins that are dangerous to children. If you smoke in another room, the toxins and fumes have been shown to be carried through walls and air ventilation systems.

If you are worried that your child is living in a polluted city or town, or is exposed to too many toxins, you can actually obtain this information from the Environmental Protection Agency (www.epa.gov). Towns, and certainly schools, that have high levels of certain air toxins are now mandated to be 'cleaned up' in order to be considered safe for children (www.epa.gov/air/caa/peg/understand.html). If you are NOT worried that your child is exposed to pollutants, cigarette smoke, excess garbage waste, or car fumes, then in the future, your child will be the one to worry, and so will his children.

TO-DO LIST: CLEAR THE AIR FOR YOUR CHILD

1. Model, model model. Lead by example. Your child will take on your behavior, without your having to say a word.

2. Talk to your child. While silent mimicking is wonderful, explain why you do what you do. And also explain that you are not perfect in any way, including in keeping the air clean. You do your best, but you often make mistakes. Children love to hear their parents' flaws! Feel free to tell them, and explain how you'll try to do better, perhaps with their help.

3. Get your child involved — teach him colors when you use different trash bins, help him pick reusable containers — let him stick on name labels, stickers, or have him decorate them with a waterproof marker.

4. Ask questions. While these are the years that 'why' questions seem to have no final answer, ask some 'why' questions of your child. Why is the gas station stinky? Why does a bird eat garbage? Why do we clean up? Why is this pond so pretty? Why is it such a clear day today?

5. Make it fun. Everything is a game for this age group. Even garbage management can be a worthwhile game.

6. Take a Deep Breath! Do it with your child. They will see how good it can feel.

Sources for Clear the Air for Your Child:

www.firstaid.about.com
www.organicconsumers.org
Clean Air, Healthy Children: Teacher's Guide and Activities for Young Children. (Wisconsin Department of Natural Resources, Bureau of Communication and Education. PO Box 7921, Madison, WI 53707. October 2004).
Capello M. "Swallow" (New Press) 2011.

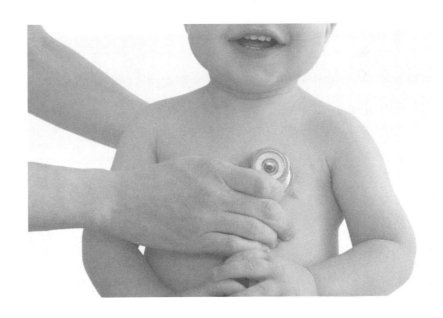

APPENDIX

GLOSSARY

Acetominophen

Commonly known by the brand name Tylenol®. Acts to reduce fever and pain. Does not require prescription.

Acral cyanosis

Blue discoloration of the palms and soles. Usually seen in young babies. Most commonly related to immature temperature regulation. However, check with doctor to make sure there is no heart or lung issue.

Adenoidectomy

Removal of adenoid tissue (lymph node tissue behind the nose).

Adenoids

Lymph node tissue that rests behind the nose. While the word is plural, there is only one, midline area of adenoid tissue.

Adenovirus

Common cold virus, which may also cause eye infections, swollen glands, fever, and sore throat.

Adrenaline

Also known as epinephrine. Medication that acts to reduce inflammation or treat severe allergic reactions. Side effects include increased heart rate and increased blood pressure. Can be administered as injection or as inhaled steam form.

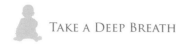

Albuterol

Medication that acts to relax and dilate lower airway passages, enabling easier breathing when wheezing or coughing is present. Usually administered in inhaled form.

Allergic Rhinitis

Chronically swollen nasal tissues due to allergies. May be associated with nasal congestion and sneezing.

Alveoli

Air-filled sacs in the lungs that help to transport oxygen to the blood.

Aminophylline

Medication used to prevent and treat wheezing by relaxing and opening air passages in the lungs. Can be given as oral or intravenous medication.

Anaphylaxis

Severe allergic reaction, associated with airway swelling of the tongue, lips, throat and/or windpipe.

Anemia

Low red blood cell count.

Anti-histamine

Medication which blocks receptors (histamine receptors) responsible for allergic reactions.

Antibiotics

Medications used to treat bacterial (not viral) infections.

Apnea of Prematurity

Periods of absent breathing, seen in premature babies. Due to immature reflexes needed to stimulate breathing.

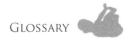

Apnea

A period of one breath cycle (five seconds in adults; three seconds in a child) during sleep where there is no breathing.

Apnea/Hypopnea Index (AHI)

Measurement of the degree of apnea one has, based on a one-night sleep study evaluation. The AHI is the average number of apneas or hypopneas one experiences in one hour of sleep. AHI of >1 is considered to be abnormal in children; AHI of >5 is considered to be abnormal in adults.

Asthma

A chronic inflammatory disorder of the airway, usually affecting the bronchi and lungs.

Attention Deficit/Hyperactivity Disorder (ADHD)

Behavioral disorder consisting of a constellation of signs and symptoms related to inattention, hyperactiviy, impulsivity, and occasionally oppositional activities.

Bacterial

Related to a micro-organism (bacteria), in reference to an illness.

Barium Swallow Study

A radiologic test to visualize swallowing function of the mouth and esophagus. The patient drinks barium, a white liquid, that can be seen on an X-ray.

Biphasic Stridor

Turbulent airflow during both breathing in and out.

Bordatella Pertussis

Bacteria which causes whooping cough (pertussis).

Bronchi

Small air passage tubes leading from the windpipe to the lungs.

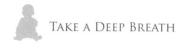

Bronchioles

Small air passages leading from the bronchi to the alveoli.

Bronchiolitis

Acute respiratory infection, commonly seen in young infants, causing inflammation of the small air passages leading to the lungs. Associated with cough, fever, and sometimes difficulty in breathing/wheezing.

Bronchodilator

Medication that acts to open up blocked or swollen air passages in the bronchi and lungs (e.g., Albuterol, Levalbuterol, Ipratropium Bromide).

Bronchopulmonary Dysplasia (BPD)

Poorly developed or immature lungs and bronchi, commonly seen in babies who are born prematurely.

Budesonide (Pulmicort®)

Inhaled liquid steroid medication that turns to steam form when administered via nebulizer. Acts to reduce airway swelling.

Caffeine

Medication used in premature infants to increase breathing frequency, decrease apnea, and minimize need for mechanical ventilation.

Carbon Dioxide

Gas that is exhaled during regular breathing.

Cardiopulmonary Resuscitation (CPR)

Breathing and heart beat support by providing mouth-to-mouth resuscitation and chest compressions to someone who is not breathing and has no heartbeat.

Central Apnea

Absence of breathing due to a neurologic (brain/nervous system) problem or immaturity. Most healthy babies have mild central apnea.

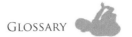

Central Sleep Apnea
> Entity whereby a person has periods of absent breathing during sleep, due to lack of appropriate brain reflexes needed to stimulate breathing.

Choanal Atresia
> A congenital disorder whereby the back part of the nasal passage is blocked by either bone or extra tissue. If this occurs on both sides of the nose, a baby cannot breathe at all without mechanical ventilation support.

Computed Tomography (CT Scan)
> Specialized X-ray used to identify problems in the sinuses or chest, when plain radiographs such as sinus X-rays or chest X-rays do not reveal the problem.

Coxsackie Virus
> Virus which can cause painful sores at the back of the throat, as well as occasionally the palms and soles. When all three are affected, the infection is called 'hand-foot-and-mouth disease'.

Croup
> Acute respiratory infection of the upper windpipe, usually caused by a type of cold virus. Swelling of the upper windpipe causes a 'barky' cough as well as difficulty in breathing. Seen most commonly in infants and toddlers.

Cyanosis
> Blue discoloration on the lips, mouth, nailbeds, or skin. A sign of low oxygen level in the blood.

Cystic Fibrosis
> Chronic inflammatory disease affecting the lungs, sinuses, and gastro-intestinal tract.

Decongestant
> Any medication, either given by mouth or as a nasal spray, which acts to shrink swollen tissues of the nose and sinuses.

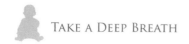

Dexamethasone (Decadron®)

Strong anti-inflammatory medication used to treat illnesses associated with airway blockage.

Diphenhydramine (Benadryl®)

Over-the-counter anti-histamine medication used for nasal congestion or allergy symptoms.

DTaP

Vaccine given as a series of booster shots throughout early infancy and childhood. Prevents Diphtheria, Tetanus, and Pertussis.

Eczema

Inflammatory skin disorder, with flaking, occasional redness, and itching. Can be seen in infants or young children. Often associated with environmental allergies.

Electrolytes

Chemicals in the body which help to regulate fluid balance (such as sodium, potassium, chloride, bicarbonate).

Enzyme

Substance in the body that acts to break down/digest ingested substances.

Eosinophils

White blood cells, when elevated, often associated with environmental allergies.

Ephedrine

A common over-the-counter cold medicine that reduces inflamed nasal passages by shrinking swollen blood vessels.

Epiglottis

The leaf-like cartilage tissue at the top of the voice box. The epiglottis protects the windpipe by closing over and protecting the voice box when one swallows,

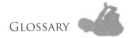

and allows for breathing and speaking by opening over the voice box when one breathes or speaks.

Epiglottitis

Acute respiratory infection of the epiglottis, usually caused by the bacteria hemophilus influenzae (H. flu). Can lead to life-threatening breathing problems. Widespread immunization against H. flu has nearly eradicated this disease.

Epinephrine

Medication given either as an inhaled form or as an injection to reduce swollen tissues by reducing swollen blood vessels. Also referred to as 'adrenaline'.

Epi-Pen

Injectible epinephrine given to severely allergic patients, to be used in the event of a severe allergic reaction or anaphylaxis.

Esophagus

The muscular tube that carries food from the mouth to the stomach. Similar in consistency to a small bicycle inner tube.

Expiratory Stridor

Turbulent airflow when breathing out.

Fifth Disease

Viral illness caused by parvovirus B19, with outbreak of the rash seen after mild cold symptoms have subsided. Classic signs are red ('slapped') cheeks, lacy rash of the trunk, arms, and legs, and rarely joint pain.

Gastroesophageal Reflux Disease (GERD)

The entity whereby reverse movement of food, liquid or stomach contents into the esophagus leads to symptoms of vomiting, discomfort, or breathing problems.

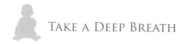

Gastroesophageal Reflux
> The reverse movement of food, liquid, or stomach contents from the stomach to the esophagus.

General Anesthesia
> Complete anesthesia, where one is asleep and unconscious. Breathing is supported by a ventilator (breathing machine).

Guaifenisen
> Cough medication used to reduce thickness of mucus produced during a cough/cold.

Hand-Foot-And-Mouth Disease
> Acute infectious illness caused by the coxsackie virus, leading to painful sores of the palms, soles, and throat. Very contagious.

Heimlich Maneuver
> Procedure utilized to extract a foreign object lodged in an individual's air passage. Does not need to be learned or performed by a medically-trained person, and can be performed on children or adults.

Hemophilus influenzae (H. flu)
> Bacteria responsible for causing such illnesses as epiglottitis, severe pneumonia, and meningitis. Vaccination against H. flu is part of the routine immunization schedule for infants and children.

Herd Immunity
> The concept that providing immunization to large communities enables eradication of the target disease in that community.

High Efficiency Particulate Air (HEPA) Filter
> Fibrous air filtration system that blocks small air pollutants from entering the air.

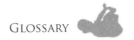

Hoarseness
Entity whereby ones voice has an irregular, or raspy quality.

Human Papillomavirus (HPV)
Virus responsible for causing genital and airway lesions (warts).

Ibuprofen
Commonly known under brand names, Motrin® or Advil®. Acts to reduce fever and pain.

Immune System
Organ system responsible for fighting infections.

Immunoglobulin E (IgE)
Substance in the bloodstream that may be elevated in the setting of environmental allergies.

Infant Botulism
A potentially life-threatening disease in which a bacteria (clostridium botulinum) grows within a baby's stomach and intestines. Can lead to loss or slowing of breathing.

Influenza
Commonly referred to as the flu, is a contagious disease caused by a virus (influenza virus).

Inspiratory Stridor
Turbulent airflow when breathing in.

Ipratropium Bromide (Atrovent®)
Inhaled medication used to prevent wheezing, coughing, and chest tightness.

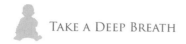

Laryngomalacia

Floppy tissue above the voice box, usually including a floppy epiglottis. Seen commonly in infants.

Laryngotracheobronchitis (LTB)

Another term for croup.

Levalbuterol (Xopenex®)

Liquid medication that becomes steam when administered via nebulizer. Acts by dilating (opening) blocked air passages in the bronchi and lungs (bronchodilator).

Lidocaine

Medication, usually given intravenously, to reduce airway activity. Also used as a local or topical numbing anesthetic medication.

Lymph Nodes

Solid masses of tissue associated with the immune system function, found throughout the body.

Lymphoid Tissue

Tissue related to the lymph nodes/immune system.

Magnetic Resonance Imaging (MRI)

Highly specialized, high-definition radiologic test, which is utilized to identify abnormalities or growths in the tissues as opposed to bones. No radiations is given.

Meningitis

Infection of the tissues lining the brain and spinal cord. Can be caused by viruses or bacteria.

Mixed Apnea

Periods of absent breathing, due to either airway blockage and/or abnormal breathing reflexes.

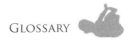

Nasal Saline

> Medication (over-the-counter) used as nasal drops, spray, or irrigation. Can be used for newborns as well. Aids in clearing nasal crusting, mucus, or blockage and helps to treat colds, congestion, and minor allergies.

Nasal Septum

> The center part of the nose, which divides the right side from the left. The front part is made of cartilage; the back part consists of bone.

Nasal Steroid Sprays

> Medications given as nasal puffs, to reduce nasal swelling in the setting of allergies or chronic nasal congestion.

Nasal Turbinates

> Liners inside the nose that help to filter dust, produce mucus, and prevent nasal crusting. When too large or inflamed, they can cause nasal congestion/sinus infections.

Nasopharynx

> Space directly behind the nose, at the upper back of the throat. The adenoids sit in the nasopharynx.

Nebulizer

> Machine which converts liquid medication to an inhalable steam form.

Neonatal Rhinitis

> 'Stuffy nose of the newborn' could be caused by either dryness, small nasal passages, respiratory illness, or undetected allergy. Treatment is usually humidification, nasal saline drops, and rarely prescription nasal drops.

Obligate Nasal Breathers

> Inability to breathe through the mouth, even without blockage. Infants under the age of three to four months are obligate nasal breathers; that is, they are unable to breathe through their mouth, and must breathe through their noses.

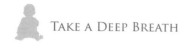

Obstructive Apnea
Absence of breathing due to a blockage in the airway.

Obstructive Sleep Apnea (OSA)
Entity whereby a person has blocked airways during sleep, leading to periods of no breathing in the setting of making an effort to breathe.

Oxymetazoline
Commonly known as Afrin® nasal spray. Acts as a nasal decongestant by reducing the size of the swollen nasal tissue. Effect is usually seen within 30 minutes. While no prescription is required, check with your doctor before giving this to your baby or child. Use no more than two sprays, two times per day, for two days.

Palivizumab (Synagis®)
Anti-viral vaccine used to prevent RSV infections in certain high-risk infants.

Parvovirus B19
Virus responsible for causing Fifth Disease.

Pertussis
Severe upper respiratory infection, commonly known as whooping cough. Coughing spells are followed by a 'whoop' sound as the patient tries to breathe in air through the swollen tissues of the throat.

pH Probe
A test to assess for Gastroesophageal Reflux Disease. A small tube is placed through the nose, down the esophagus. It is usually left in place for 24 hours, and measures the pH of the contents of the esophagus. Low pH indicates acidity, and likelihood of GERD.

Phenylephrine
Nasal decongestant used for colds, allergies, or sinus pressure. Usually an ingredient in over-the-counter cold medicine preparations.

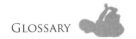

Plagiocephaly
Flattening of the back or side of a newborn's head, most commonly associated with sleeping on ones back. Usually is temporary, and rarely requires intervention.

Pneumonia
A respiratory infection involving one or both lungs. May be caused by either a virus or a bacteria.

Prednisone
Strong anti-inflammatory medication with multiple uses, including to reduce airway swelling.

Pseudoephedrine
A common over-the-counter cold medicine that reduces swollen nasal passages by shrinking swollen blood vessels.

Pulmonary Function Tests
Tests of lung function, whereby the patient exhales and inhales through tubes. Amount of airflow and degree of obstruction or restriction are recorded on meters, based on lung capacity and function.

RadioAllergoSorbent Test (RAST)
Blood test which determines the degree of allergic response to a given allergen.

Reactive Airway Disease
Entity whereby the bronchi or lungs become inflamed or irritated during respiratory illnesses or allergic stimulants.

Rebound Response
The event where the over-use of a medication causes the reverse effect from that desired.

Recurrent Respiratory Papillomatosis (RRP)
Disease entity, most commonly seen in children, caused by HPV. Results in 'warts' of the voicebox and/or windpipe, with associated hoarseness and breathing difficulty.

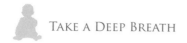

Respiratory Syncytial Virus (RSV)

A very common virus that leads to mild, cold-like symptoms in adults and older healthy children. RSV infections in young babies are more serious, and may lead to bronchitis or pneumonia, especially in those who are born prematurely.

Retraction

Inward and outward muscle movement of the lower neck, between the ribs, or stomach, indicating breathing difficulty.

Rheumatic Fever

Inflammatory disease that may develop after an infection with Streptococcus, such as strep throat or scarlet fever. Can affect the heart, joints, skin, and brain.

Rhinovirus

The most common virus causing a cold.

Ribavirin

Anti-viral drug used in treating severe RSV (respiratory syncitial virus) infections.

Roseola/Exanthem Subitum/Sixth Disease

Rash commonly seen in infants, with fever and cold symptoms.

Scarlet Fever

Severe infection secondary to a Streptococcal infection, with 'sand-paper'-type rash, sore throat, and high fever.

Screamers Nodules

Small bumps that form on the vocal cords of people (classically children) who overuse their voice. Nodules result in hoarseness and breathiness when speaking.

Sleep Medicine

Medical specialty focusing on evaluation and treatment of sleep disorders. Sleep Medicine specialists may be neurologists, pulmonologists, or otolaryngologists.

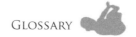

Sleep Study/Polysomnogram

Test performed during one night of sleep, measuring such parameters as oxygen levels and presence or absence of episodes of apnea, how long these episodes last, and how often they occur.

Soft Palate

The area of muscle tissue just behind the roof of the mouth. Important for speech and swallowing. If it's too floppy, may cause noisy breathing or snoring.

Sphincter

Rings of tight muscle tissue, which remain closed at rest, but open up with increased muscle activity.

Steroids

Strong anti-inflammatory medications, which can be given in oral form, intravenous form (into a vein), intramuscular form (as an injection), or inhaled form into the nose or chest. Must be administered by prescription, under a doctor's supervision. Oral and inhaled forms may be administered at home.

Streptococcus

Bacteria responsible for illnesses such as tonsillitis, bronchitis, ear infections, and pneumonia.

Stridor

Turbulent airflow, anywhere from the voicebox to the windpipe. Usually heard as a high-pitched, squeaky sound.

Suction Catheters

Tiny straw-like tubes that suction secretions such as mucus, saliva, or phlegm from the back of the nose or mouth. Very commonly used in delivery rooms or newborn care units to clear babies' air passages.

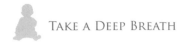

Sudden Infant Death Syndrome (SIDS)
> The leading cause of death in infants between ages 1–12 months. Most common in infants between 2–4 months. Unexplained death during sleep, thought to be due to blocked or insufficient breathing.

Surfactant
> Substance produced by newborn lungs, enabling them to fill with air after birth.

Sutures (cranial)
> Spaces separating the bones of the skull. These sutures allow for brain growth during the first 6 to 12 months of life.

Sweat Chloride Test
> Skin test used to test amount of chloride ion in sweat. Abnormal levels are an indication of cystic fibrosis diagnosis.

Tamiflu®/Relenza®
> Prescription medications which act to reduce the duration of symptoms secondary to influenza.

TDaP
> Booster form of vaccine preventing Tetanus, Diphtheria, and Pertussis. Given to older children and adults.

Tonsils
> Lymph node tissue that rests at the back of the mouth, one on each side.

Trachea
> The windpipe. Between the voice box and the bronchus. The consistency of a partially-inflated bicycle tire.

Tracheomalacia
> Floppiness of the trachea (windpipe), caused by either intrinsic cartilage weakness or from extrinsic compression.

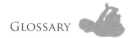

Turbinate Reduction
Procedure which shrinks swollen nasal turbinates to improve nasal breathing.

Vasomotor Rhinitis
Chronic nasal swelling/congestion not caused by allergies.

Ventilation
Breathing in and out. Mechanical ventilation is providing breathing via breathing machine, through a breathing tube which is inserted into the windpipe.

Vocal Nodules
Small benign growths on the vocal cords, commonly seen in individuals who strain or overuse their voice. Result is a hoarse, breathy quality when speaking.

Voice Box (Larynx)
The part of the throat which is responsible for sound. Contains the vocal cords. The top-most part of the windpipe is the larynx.

Voice Therapy
Behavioral treatment by a specialized voice therapist, with goals to 'retrain' how to use ones voice appropriately, eventually enabling vocal nodules or screamer's nodules to heal.

Wheezing
Noisy breathing due to blockage in the bronchi or lungs.

X-ray
Radiograph which shows air, bone, and soft tissue shadows.

Vaccine Recommendations

Vaccine Recommendation Schedule, Ages Zero to Six Years
(United States, 2010)
(www.cdc.gov/vaccines/recs/acip)

Birth:

Hepatitis B (HepB) (second dose between one and two months)

Two months:

Hepatitis B (if second dose is not given at one month)

Rotavirus (RV)

Diphtheria, Tetanus, Pertussis (DTaP)

Hemophilus influenzae type B (Hib)

Pneumococcal (PCV)

Inactivated Poliovirus (IPV)

Four months:

Rotavirus (RV)

Diphtheria, Tetanus, Pertussis (DTaP)

Hemophilus influenzae type B (Hib)

Pneumococcal (PCV)

Inactivated Poliovirus (IPV)

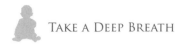

Six months:

Hepatitis B (HepB) (third dose may be given between six and 18 months)

Rotavirus (RV)

Diphtheria, Tetanus, Pertussis (DTaP)

Hemophilus influenzae type B (Hib)

Pneumococcal (PCV)

Inactivated Poliovirus (IPV) (third dose may be given between six and 18 months)

Influenza (Flu vaccine) (Yearly) (First dose must be given as two separate vaccines, one month apart)

12 months:

Hepatitis B (HepB) (if not given at six months)

Hemophilus influenzae type b (Hib) (fourth dose may be given between 12 and 15 months)

Pneumococcal (PCV)

Inactivated Poliovirus (IPV) (if not given at six months)

Influenza (Flu vaccine) (yearly)

Measles, Mumps, Rubella (MMR) (may be given between 12 and 15 months)

Varicella (may be given between 12 and 15 months)

15 months:

Hepatitis B (HepB) (if not given at six or 12 months)

Diphtheria, Tetanus, Pertussis (DTaP) (fourth dose may be given between 15 and 18 months)

Hemophilus influenzae type B (Hib) (if not given at 12 months)

Pneumococcal (PCV) (if not given at 12 months)

Inactivated Poliovirus (IPV) (if not given at six or 12 months)

Influenzae (flu vaccine) (yearly)

Measles, Mumps, Rubella (MMR) (if not given at 12 months)

Varicella (if not given at 12 months)

Hepatitis A (Hep A) (two doses between 12 and 23 months)

18 months:

Diptheria, Tetanus, Pertussis (DTaP) (if not given at 15 months)

Inactivated Poliovirus (IPV) (if not given at six, 12, or 15 months)

Influenza (Flu vaccine) (yearly)

Hepatitis A (Hep A) (two doses between 12 and 23 months)

19–23 months:

Influenza (flu vaccine) (yearly)

Hepatitis A (Hep A) (two doses between 12 and 23 months)

2–3 years:

Pneumococcal Polysaccharide Vaccine (PPSV) (for children with underlying medical conditions) (discuss with your doctor)

Influenza (Flu vaccine) (yearly)

Hepatitis A (Hep A) (for children at increased risk for infection) (discuss with your doctor)

Meningococcal vaccine (MCV) (for children with chronic immune system disease) (discuss with your doctor)

4-6 years:

Diphtheria, Tetanus, Pertussis (DTaP)

Inactivated Poliovirus (IPV)

Measles, Mumps, Rubella (MMR) (doctor may check blood levels — if adequate immunity, may hold off on this booster)

Influenza (flu vaccine) (yearly)

Varicella booster

CPR for Infants and Children

CPR for Infants from Newborn to 12 Months*

❖ If your baby is not breathing and you cannot see or feel an object blocking his throat, you will need to begin CPR.

❖ If there is another person around, ask him to call 911 and explain the situation and your location.

❖ If you are by yourself, begin CPR and then call 911 after two minutes of performing CPR.

❖ First, place your baby flat, face-up, on a firm surface such as on a carpeted or hard floor. Do not place him on a bed, couch, chair, or table.

❖ Tilt his neck back gently, lifting his chin in the upward direction.

❖ Put your mouth over your baby's nose and mouth and give two small breaths. Remember, your baby's lungs are much smaller than yours, and you do not need to give large breaths.

❖ If there is no breathing (crying or coughing equals breathing), give 30 chest compressions.

❖ To give a baby chest compressions, place your second and third finger about three finger-breadths (one to two inches) below his nipples in the center of his chest.

❖ Each chest compression should be quick, and you should compress about half to one inch down with each compression.

❖ Give one to two compressions every second (about 100 per minute).

❖ Continue this cycle of two breaths/30 chest compressions until help arrives.

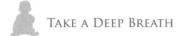

❖ Before giving a breath, check your baby's mouth to see if you can see a dislodged object. If you can see it, grab it and remove it. If he is still not breathing, continue CPR. If he vomits, turn his head to the side, to help clear the vomit from his mouth.

❖ After two minutes of CPR (about two to three cycles of breaths and compressions), call 911 if you are by yourself.

❖ Resume CPR, and follow the instructions of the 911 operator after you complete the call.

❖ Even if your baby resumes breathing, you still need to call 911 if you have given CPR at all.

---

*According to the American Heart Association, it is now recommended that CPR for adults should begin with chest compressions only, not breathing support, as most adults who require CPR are suffering from a heart-related event. However, the vast majority of children who require CPR have a breathing problem and not a heart problem. Therefore, breathing support and treatment is still recommended for children who need CPR. It is strongly recommended that all parents, parents-to-be, and caregivers take a CPR course (as well as refresher courses at least once per year). These are given at local hospitals, some schools, and at local American Red Cross chapters (www.redcross.org), 1-800-627-7000.

CPR for Children Over One Year

❖ If you are alone with your child, and she is not breathing, begin CPR. Continue CPR for two minutes, and then call 911.

❖ If you are not alone, begin CPR and ask someone to call 911.

❖ Place your child lying down with face up, on a hard surface.

❖ Do not place her on a bed, chair, couch, or table. The floor or the ground is best.

❖ Check your child's mouth for an object. If you can see it, remove it.

❖ If you cannot see an object, and/or there is still no breathing, give two breaths.

❖ To give breaths, gently tilt your child's neck up, with her chin in the upward position. Pinch her nose closed with your fingers, and give two small breaths. Remember, your child's lungs are smaller than yours, so small breaths are adequate.

❖ If your child does not begin breathing, coughing, or crying, place the palm portion of your hand (the part just before your wrist) in the middle of her breastbone, between her nipples to give chest compressions.

❖ Push down quickly, about two inches, and let the chest come back up. Do this 30 times, at a rate of about two compressions per second (100 times per minute).

❖ If there is still no breathing, crying, or coughing, give two breaths again.

❖ Continue this, alternating between breaths and chest compressions, until help arrives.

❖ Even if your child resumes breathing, you still need to call 911 if CPR was needed at all.

Index

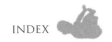

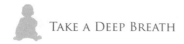

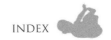

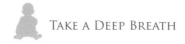

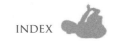